HUMAN SKIN CANCER, POTENTIAL BIOMARKERS AND THERAPEUTIC TARGETS

Edited by **Miroslav Blumenberg**

Human Skin Cancer, Potential Biomarkers and Therapeutic Targets
http://dx.doi.org/10.5772/61922
Edited by Miroslav Blumenberg

Contributors

Małgorzata Przybyło, Marcelina Janik, Dorota Hoja-Łukowicz, Ewa Pocheć, Anna Lityńska, Robert Rollins, Kimberly Kim, Cheng-Chung Tsao, Mandi Murph, Ali Alshamrani, James Franklin, Aaron Beedle, Miroslav Blumenberg

Published by InTech

Janeza Trdine 9, 51000 Rijeka, Croatia

Publishing Process Manager Romina Rovan
Technical Editor SPi Global
Cover InTech Design team

First published October, 2016
Printed in Croatia

Additional hard copies can be obtained from orders@intechopen.com

Human Skin Cancer, Potential Biomarkers and Therapeutic Targets, Edited by Miroslav Blumenberg
p. cm.
Print ISBN 978-953-51-2710-9
Online ISBN 978-953-51-2711-6

For EU product safety concerns:
IN TECH d.o.o., Prolaz Marije Krucifikse Kozulić 3, 51000 Rijeka, Croatia,
info@intechopen.com or visit our website at intechopen.com.

Meet the editor

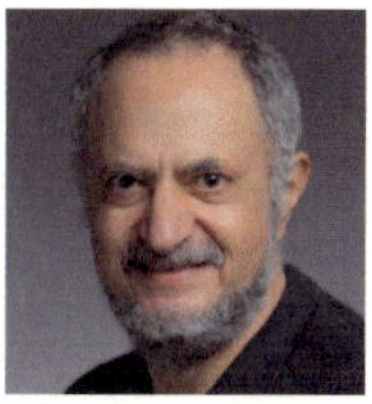

Miroslav Blumenberg, PhD, was born in Subotica and received his BSc in Belgrade, Yugoslavia. He completed his PhD in organic chemistry at MIT; he followed this up with two postdoctoral study periods at Stanford University. Since 1983, he has been a faculty member of the R.O. Perelman Department of Dermatology, NYU School of Medicine, where he is a codirector of a training grant in cutaneous biology. Dr Blumenberg's research is focused on the epidermis, expression of keratin genes, transcription profiling, keratinocyte differentiation, inflammatory diseases and cancers, and, most recently, the effects of the microbiome on the skin. He has published over 100 peer-reviewed research articles and graduated numerous PhD and postdoctoral students. Dr Blumenberg lives in New York, USA, with his wife and two children.

Contents

Preface IX

Section 1 Introduction 1

Chapter 1 **Introductory Chapter: A Short Primer on Human Skin Cancers 3**
Miroslav Blumenberg

Section 2 Epigenetics 7

Chapter 2 **The Emerging Epigenetic Landscape in Melanoma 9**
Robert A. Rollins, Kimberly H. Kim and Cheng-Chung Tsao

Section 3 Cell Surface Markers 39

Chapter 3 **Glycosylation of Integrins in Melanoma Progression 41**
Ewa Pocheć and Anna Lityńska

Chapter 4 **Bitter Sweetness of Malignant Melanoma: Deciphering the Role of Cell Surface Glycosylation in Tumour Progression and Metastasis 63**
Małgorzata Przybyło, Marcelina E. Janik and Dorota Hoja-Łukowicz

Chapter 5 **Cadherins and their Role in Malignant Transformation: Implications for Skin Cancer Progression 89**
Marcelina E. Janik, Dorota Hoja-Łukowicz and Małgorzata Przybyło

Section 4 Metabolism 123

Chapter 6 **Inhibiting Lactate Dehydrogenase A Enhances the Cytotoxicity of the Mitochondria Accumulating Antioxidant, Mitoquinone, in Melanoma Cells 125**
Ali A. Alshamrani, James L. Franklin, Aaron M. Beedle and Mandi M. Murph

Preface

Skin cancers constitute arguably the most common and increasingly prevalent human neoplasms. The most common human skin cancers are basal cell carcinomas (BCCs) and squamous cell carcinomas (SCCs), but the most serious and most often fatal are malignant melanomas (MMs) and Merkel cell carcinomas (MCCs). In this volume most chapters, understandably, deal with melanoma, the deadliest of skin cancers, and in particular with the cell surface proteins, potential melanoma markers {Mason, 1996, #3609}.

In the chapter "The Emerging Epigenetic Landscape in Melanoma," Rollins et al. discuss the epigenetic changes in DNA and chromatin, which are increasingly associated with this cancer. The authors review the epigenetic changes potentially involved, depict the interplay between epigenetic and genetic factors, and go on to propose potential therapeutic approaches to target the epigenetic changes in MM.

Several of the chapters in this volume focus on the posttranscriptional modification of the proteins at the melanocyte cell surface and their role in tumorigenesis and potential as therapeutic targets. Specifically, in the chapter "Glycosylation of Integrins in Melanoma Progression," Pocheć and Lityńska describe the posttranscriptional extracellular modifications of integrins, modifications associated with melanoma progression. Integrin modifications are particularly important because integrins both mediate adhesion of melanocytes to their extracellular matrix and inform the cells about their environment; changes in integrin glycans can have profound roles in invasion and metastasis of melanoma. M. Przybyło in "Bitter Sweetness of Malignant Melanoma" focuses on the role of glycosylation of the cell surface proteins in MM progression and metastasis, suggesting a role of glycan changes in increased cell motility and hence higher invasive and metastatic potential. Similar theme is the focus of the chapter "Cadherins and Their Role in Malignant Transformation: Implications for Skin Cancer Progression" by Janik et al. Cadherins are transmembrane adhesion proteins. The changes of cadherin glycosylation occur in skin cancers, both carcinomas and melanomas.

In a very interesting approach, A. Alshamrani et al. describe a potential to target the mitochondria of melanoma cells. In the chapter "Inhibiting Lactate Dehydrogenase A Enhances the Cytotoxicity of the Mitochondria-Accumulating Antioxidant, Mitoquinone, in Melanoma Cells," the authors investigate the mitochondria-targeting antioxidant mitoquinone, alone or in combination with other cancer-fighting drugs. Alshamrani et al. show its effectiveness especially in melanoma cells with wild-type BRAF.

In conclusion, this volume presents various aspects of human skin cancers, their mechanisms of formation, their potential biomarkers, and their therapeutic targets, a component of the large worldwide effort to combat and eradicate this growing health concern.

Miroslav Blumenberg
NYU Langone Medical Center,
New York, USA

Section 1

Introduction

Chapter 1

Introductory Chapter: A Short Primer on Human Skin Cancers

Miroslav Blumenberg

Additional information is available at the end of the chapter

http://dx.doi.org/10.5772/65356

Skin cancers constitute arguably the most common and increasingly prevalent human neoplasms. In United States alone, it is estimated that 76,400 patients will develop melanoma and 10,100 will die from the disease [1]. Several risk factors, ultraviolet light the most important of these, but also environmental carcinogens, contribute to the increasing incidence of skin cancers, especially among light-skinned individuals [2]. The most common human skin cancers are basal cell carcinoma (BCC) and squamous cell carcinoma (SCC), but the most serious and most often fatal are malignant melanoma (MM) and Merkel cell carcinoma (MCC) [3].

Basal cell carcinoma is the most common type of skin cancer, caused by ultraviolet (UV) light, specifically UV-B, and its incidence increases with age. Most commonly, it occurs on sun-exposed areas, such as the face, neck, scalp, forearms, hands, legs and feet. Usually, it is a slowly growing, very rarely metastasizing, locally destructive tumor, which, if ignored, may invade the underlying tissues, bone or cartilage [4].

Basal cell carcinomas arise in keratinocyte stem cells [5]. Usually, in BCCs, the hedgehog signaling pathway is activated causing neoplastic transformation of keratinocytes. Signaling by smoothened, via the cognate receptors, activates the hedgehog signaling pathway and has been implicated in BCC pathogenesis [6].

The most common treatment for BCC is surgical excision, nowadays using Mohs micrographic surgery to ensure complete excision while sparing the surrounding tissue [4]. Curettage, cryotherapy or laser ablation is sometimes used for lesions considered less risky.

Squamous cell carcinoma is the second most common skin cancer worldwide. It usually occurs in sun-exposed areas, frequently on lips, forehead and scalp, ears and pre-auricular regions, but can occur anywhere on skin [7]. It can both invade locally and can metastasize. Chronic sun exposure is the main risk factor for SCC occurrence. Human papillomaviruses and exposure to carcinogens, such as arsenic or polycyclic aromatic hydrocarbons, are contributing risk factors. Transplant recipients and other immunosuppressed patients are at significantly increased risk for SCC [8].

The appearance of SSCs is variable, and it may present as an ulcer, lump or red patch on the skin, often with scaling or crusting. It is common in elderly. Actinic or solar keratosis, caused by exposure to UV light, is a premalignant lesion, a risk factor potentially leading to progression to invasive SCC. SCCs starting within actinic keratosis are generally low risk, with a more favorable prognosis [7].

Squamous cell carcinoma is usually surgically excised, using Mohs micrographic surgery, with chemotherapy including cisplatin or 5-fluorouracil less common [4]. Actinic keratoses may be treated as a prevention modality for SCC.

Merkel cell carcinoma is a rare but very aggressive primary skin cancer with high mortality rate [9]. While ultraviolet light and immunosuppression seem to have a role in causing MCC, association has been established with Merkel cell polyomavirus [10]. MCC appears as a rapidly growing lesion, usually on the head and neck skin. It quickly proceeds to metastasize, locally and distantly. It is treated with aggressive surgery, but the survival rates are poor.

Malignant melanoma is by far the deadliest of skin cancers! MM is highly invasive locally and, unfortunately, has a high propensity to metastasize [11, 12]. It is usually recognized as a new or newly changed lesion on the skin. Flat superficial spreading form of MM can appear in a variety of colors, from black or blue to brown, gray, pink or white. The nodular form of MMs is usually darkly pigmented and asymmetrical, and sometimes poorly differentiated, unpigmented to appear amelanotic, pink or red. Lentigo maligna melanoma develops on sun-exposed skin in the elderly, slowly enlarging over several years.

Melanoma is a malignant neoplasm of melanocytes, not keratinocytes. The main risk factor is UV light, especially UV-B, and both occasional severe sunburn and chronic sun exposure have been associated with MM formation [13]. People who burn easily, with light skin, blue eyes, red hair and freckles are at increased risk of MM. Giant congenital melanocytic nevi present a high risk, although MM can arise within pre-existing benign melanotic nevi or in normal appearing skin. MM can appear at any site, on skin as well as on oral, genital, urinary or ocular epithelial surfaces.

Population is urged to use the ABCDE rule when ascertaining the presence of MM [14]. These stand for A—asymmetry of the lesion, B—border (irregular), C—color (non-uniform), D—diameter (>6 mm, size of a pencil eraser) and E—evolving (changing in size, shape, color etc.). These features should raise apprehension of MM.

Wide local excision of the area of diagnosis is required. A sentinel lymph node biopsy is performed often, and whole body CT and PET scan are used occasionally in search for metastases. Conventional chemotherapy generally does not work. Recent research into mutations associated with MM identified BRAF gene as frequently mutated [15]; this led to development of specific inhibitors of the corresponding signal transduction pathways such as

Vemurafenib, specifically targeting a recurrent mutation in BRAF, or Imatinib, a more general tyrosine kinase inhibitor [16]. Ipilimumab, a monoclonal antibody blocking CTLA-4, enhances immunotherapy against MM. Prognosis depends very much on the stage at which the tumor is detected.

In this volume, most chapters, understandably, deal with melanoma, the deadliest of skin cancers, and in particular with the cell surface proteins, potential melanoma markers [17].

In conclusion, this volume presents various aspects of human skin cancers, their mechanisms of formation, potential biomarkers and therapeutic targets, a component of the large world-wide effort to combat and eradicate this growing health concern.

Author details

Miroslav Blumenberg

Address all correspondence to: miroslav.blumenberg@nyumc.org

The R.O.Perelman Department of Dermatology and Department of Biochemistry and Molecular Pharmacology, NYU Langone Medical Center, New York, USA

References

[1] Bibbins-Domingo K, Grossman DC, Curry SJ, Davidson KW, Ebell M, Epling JW, Jr., et al. Screening for skin cancer: US Preventive Services Task Force Recommendation Statement. JAMA. 2016;316:429–435.

[2] Leiter U, Eigentler T, Garbe C. Epidemiology of skin cancer. Adv Exp Med Biol. 2014;810:120–140.

[3] Gordon R. Skin cancer: an overview of epidemiology and risk factors. Semin Oncol Nurs. 2013;29:160–169.

[4] Kauvar AN, Cronin T, Jr., Roenigk R, Hruza G, Bennett R. Consensus for nonmelanoma skin cancer treatment: basal cell carcinoma, including a cost analysis of treatment methods. Dermatol Surg. 2015;41:550–571.

[5] Song IY, Balmain A. Cellular reprogramming in skin cancer. Semin Cancer Biol. 2015;32:32–39.

[6] Otsuka A, Levesque MP, Dummer R, Kabashima K. Hedgehog signaling in basal cell carcinoma. J Dermatol Sci. 2015;78:95–100.

[7] Stratigos A, Garbe C, Lebbe C, Malvehy J, del Marmol V, Pehamberger H, et al. Diagnosis and treatment of invasive squamous cell carcinoma of the skin:

European consensus-based interdisciplinary guideline. Eur J Cancer. 2015;51:1989–2007.

[8] Kim C, Cheng J, Colegio OR. Cutaneous squamous cell carcinomas in solid organ transplant recipients: emerging strategies for surveillance, staging, and treatment. Semin Oncol. 2016;43:390–394.

[9] Verzi AE, Amin SM, Guitart J, Micali G. Merkel cell carcinoma: a review. G Ital Dermatol Venereol. 2015;150:419–428.

[10] Grundhoff A, Fischer N. Merkel cell polyomavirus, a highly prevalent virus with tumorigenic potential. Curr Opin Virol. 2015;14:129–137.

[11] Wong DJ, Ribas A. Targeted therapy for melanoma. Cancer Treat Res. 2016;167:251–262.

[12] Gruber F, Kastelan M, Brajac I, Saftic M, Peharda V, Cabrijan L, et al. Molecular and genetic mechanisms in melanoma. Coll Antropol. 2008;32(Suppl 2):147–152.

[13] Chang C, Murzaku EC, Penn L, Abbasi NR, Davis PD, Berwick M, et al. More skin, more sun, more tan, more melanoma. Am J Public Health. 2014;104:e92–e99.

[14] Benelli C, Roscetti E, Dal Pozzo V. Reproducibility of the clinical criteria (ABCDE rule) and dermatoscopic features (7FFM) for the diagnosis of malignant melanoma. Eur J Dermatol. 2001;11:234–239.

[15] Criscito MC, Polsky D, Stein JA. The genetic evolution of melanoma. N Engl J Med. 2016;374:993.

[16] Zakrzewski J, Geraghty LN, Rose AE, Christos PJ, Mazumdar M, Polsky D, et al. Clinical variables and primary tumor characteristics predictive of the development of melanoma brain metastases and post-brain metastases survival. Cancer. 2011;117:1711–1720.

[17] Mason MD, Allman R, Quibell M. Adhesion molecules in melanoma—more than just superglue? J R Soc Med. 1996;89:393–395.

Section 2

Epigenetics

Chapter 2

The Emerging Epigenetic Landscape in Melanoma

Robert A. Rollins, Kimberly H. Kim and
Cheng-Chung Tsao

Additional information is available at the end of the chapter

http://dx.doi.org/10.5772/64733

Abstract

Melanoma is the deadliest form of skin cancer. The disease is driven by molecular alterations in oncogenic signaling pathways, such as mitogen-activated protein kinase (MAPK) and phosphatidylinositol 3-kinase (PI3K). Activating mutations in oncogenes, such as *BRAF* and *NRAS*, and inactivating mutations in tumor suppressors genes, such as *PTEN*, promote this disease by altering cellular processes involved in growth, survival, and migration. Therapies targeting critical nodes in these pathways have demonstrated efficacy in clinical trials, but their therapeutic potential has been limited by the rapid onset of drug resistance. Durable therapeutic responses have also been observed in patients receiving immunotherapy. However, this activity appears to be confined to a subset of patients, and combinations with targeted therapies have raised safety concerns. Accumulating evidence strongly suggests that the pathogenesis of melanoma is also shaped by the aberrant activity of epigenetic factors that regulate gene expression through the modification of DNA and chromatin. This chapter provides a comprehensive review of the epigenetic alterations in melanoma and highlights the roles played by specific chromatin regulators during disease progression. We also discuss the clinical utility of both first and second generation epigenetic therapies in the melanoma setting, placing emphasis on the potential to overcome resistance to targeted therapies and to serve as priming agents for immunotherapies.

Keywords: melanoma, epigenetics, chromatin structure, epigenetic therapy

1. Introduction

Melanoma is the most deadly form of skin cancer. While melanoma patients represent a small percentage (~1%) of the total number of skin cancer cases, this aggressive disease is responsible for the vast majority of skin cancer deaths [1]. The incidence of melanoma has been rising steadily for several decades, with a 1.4% increase in the number of new cases each year for the last 10 years. The overall 5-year survival rate is >90%, due in large part to early detection and the ability to surgically excise localized cancer cells. However, for patients with metastatic melanoma, the 5-year survival rate drops dramatically to ~17%. In 2016, it is estimated that there will be 76,380 new melanoma cases and 10,130 melanoma-related deaths, underscoring the need for therapeutic strategies to treat this disease [2].

Melanoma arises from the malignant transformation of melanocytes in the epidermal layer of the skin. During embryonic development, neural crest cells migrate from the neural tube to the skin where they give rise to melanocytes [3]. The transformation of melanocytes to melanoma is driven by oncogenic signaling pathways that are triggered by genetic and environmental factors. Metastatic melanoma cells are highly invasive and display stem cell–like properties that are characteristic of their neural crest progenitors, making them extremely aggressive and difficult to treat [4].

Therapeutic intervention in melanoma has historically focused on targeting nodes in the MAPK pathway [5]. Activating oncogenic mutations in *BRAF* and *NRAS* have been identified in 40–60% and 15–20% of melanoma patients, respectively, leading to constitutive pathway signaling that promotes cell proliferation and survival [6, 7]. While NRAS has proven extremely difficult to target pharmacologically, potent and selective small molecule inhibitors of BRAF (vemurafenib and dabrafenib) and MEK (trametinib), a downstream signaling kinase, have been approved by the FDA for the treatment of patients with metastatic melanoma harboring $BRAF^{V600}$ mutations [8–12]. While response rates in the clinic have been impressive, resistance develops quickly and in some cases these agents have been shown to exacerbate the aggressive nature of the disease due to the paradoxical activation of the MAPK pathway in cells harboring wild-type BRAF [13, 14]. The combination of BRAF and MEK inhibitors has demonstrated improved rates of progression-free survival, however, these combinations are still prone to resistance, thereby limiting the long-term survival in melanoma patients harboring $BRAFV^{600}$ mutations [15–17]. More recently, durable clinical responses have been observed following treatment with antibodies that target immune checkpoint molecules, such as PD-1 (pembrolizumab and nivolumab) and CTLA-4 (ipilimumab) [18–20]. However, the benefit of these therapies appears to be limited to smaller subsets of the overall patient population and there are potential safety concerns around the use of these agents in combination with inhibitors of the MAPK pathway [21, 22].

While recent clinical advances provide much needed hope for melanoma patients, there is a clear need to understand additional mechanisms that contribute to the pathology of this disease. To this end, emerging data has demonstrated the importance of aberrant epigenetic regulation during melanoma growth, metastasis, and drug resistance. In addition to contributing to a more thorough understanding of melanoma pathogenesis, these studies have revealed potential drug targets implicated in the regulation of chromatin structure and gene expression [23–25].

2. Epigenetic changes as a hallmark of cancer

Epigenetics is defined as heritable changes in gene expression that occur in the absence of alteration in the DNA sequence (i.e. mutations) [26]. Epigenetic regulators are enzymes and proteins that covalently modify or bind to DNA and histones to alter chromatin structure and function. These proteins are divided into three broad classes: writers, erasers, and readers. Writers and erasers are enzymes that add and remove covalent modifications, such as acetylation, methylation, and phosphorylation, while reader molecules recognize these marks and serve as downstream effector molecules [27, 28]. The combination of DNA and histone modifications and DNA- and histone-binding proteins creates an epigenetic code that governs genome-wide transcriptional networks. Epigenetic mechanisms drive gene expression programs that regulate a multitude of cellular processes, including differentiation, proliferation, pluripotency, cell migration/motility, cell signaling, and immune recognition/response [29].

The advent of next-generation sequencing (NGS) and epigenome mapping technologies has facilitated the systematic evaluation of cancer genomes. These studies have revealed a remarkably high frequency of genetic alterations in genes encoding epigenetic regulators [30, 31]. For example, genes encoding subunits of the SWI/SNF chromatin remodeling complex are mutated in 20% of all tumors, making it the second highest mutational frequency behind *TP53* [32]. In concordance with the spectrum of genetic lesions, genome-wide analysis of DNA and chromatin structure has revealed alterations in the normal patterns of DNA methylation and histone modifications [33, 34]. These epigenetic abnormalities reprogram cancer cells by altering transcriptional programs and influencing cell fate decisions and cellular identity [35]. Based on the multitude of biological pathways influenced by epigenetic reprogramming in tumors, it has been suggested that defects in epigenetic control contribute to all of the classical hallmarks of cancer [29].

3. Epigenetic alterations in melanoma

3.1. DNA methylation

In mammalian genomes, DNA methylation occurs almost exclusively in the context of 5′-CpG dinucleotides (CpGs). Hypermethylation of CpG island promoters is a common event in cancer and results in the aberrant silencing of tumor suppressor genes [36, 37]. Paradoxically, tumors are also characterized by DNA hypomethylation, primarily at repetitive DNA sequences, transposable elements, and some single-copy genes [38]. The global loss of DNA methylation is thought to promote tumorigenesis by several mechanisms, including the creation of genomic instability, the reactivation of latent retrotransposons, and the potential activation of proto-oncogenes [39].

Aberrant DNA methylation is a hallmark of malignant melanoma [40]. Hypermethylation has been observed at key tumor suppressor genes, such as *p16/INK4A*, *p14/ARF*, *RASSF1A*, and

RARβ2, and a CpG island methylator phenotype has been correlated with disease progression [40, 41]. Interestingly, the loss of methylation at repetitive elements and the hypomethylation-induced expression of cancer-testis antigens, such as *MAGE*, have also been described as markers of poor prognosis, highlighting the complexity of tumor-associated DNA methylation patterns [40, 42]. Multiple studies have also described links between DNA methylation abnormalities and $BRAF^{V600E}$-mediated signaling [43, 44]. Genome-wide epigenomic profiling of metastatic melanoma tumors has identified subgroups of patients with distinct DNA methylation patterns that correlate with specific proliferative and immune gene expression signatures and various clinical outcomes [45, 46]. In addition to the potential use as clinical biomarkers, the data suggests that the reversion of DNA methylation patterns may provide a therapeutic benefit in melanoma patients.

3.2. Histone modifications

In addition to DNA methylation, posttranslational modifications on histone tails provide another layer of epigenetic regulation. Histone deacetylases (HDAC) are highly expressed in melanoma cells and altered histone acetylation has been linked to the downregulation of tumor suppressor genes, such as *p14/ARF* and *p16/INK4a* [25, 47, 48]. In addition to changes in histone acetylation, genomic, proteomic, and immunohistochemical approaches have also identified aberrant histone methylation patterns [49–51]. The advent of genome-wide chromatin immunoprecipitation has also uncovered global redistribution of histone marks, such as methylation on lysine 27 of histone H3 (H3K27me) [52, 53]. These observations suggest that histone modifications cooperate with DNA methylation to reprogram gene expression patterns during melanoma progression. They also point toward underlying defects in the enzymes and proteins that regulate these epigenetic mechanisms.

4. Genetic landscape of epigenetic regulators in melanoma

The emergence of NGS has proven to be a powerful tool in identifying oncogenic driver mutations. In 2012, two independent studies reported whole-genome sequencing data from 121 and 147 primary melanoma tumors, respectively [54, 55]. In addition to confirming a high frequency of oncogenic mutations in the *BRAF* and *NRAS* genes, these studies identified loss-of-function mutations in the SWI/SNF components *ARID2, ARID1A, ARID1B*, and *SMARCA4* as well as hot-spot mutations in the histone methyltransferase EZH2 [54, 55]. Identical *EZH2 Y641* mutations had previously been identified in germinal center diffuse large B cell lymphoma (DLBCL) and follicular lymphoma (FL) where they have been shown to result in gain-of-function activity [56, 57].

The high frequency of mutations in epigenetic regulators was recently confirmed in an NGS analysis of 38 treatment-naive melanoma samples [23]. Targeted sequencing of 275 known cancer genes revealed mutations in genes encoding known epigenetic regulators, including histone methyltransferases (*MLL2, SETD2*), chromatin remodeling factors (*ARID1B, ARID2*), and DNA demethylases (*TET2*). Interestingly, 92.1% of the patient melanoma samples harbored at least one mutation in an epigenetic regulator and UVB-signature mutations were found more commonly among epigenetic genes.

Analysis of publicly available data from The Cancer Genome Atlas (TCGA) confirms the high frequency of genetic lesions in epigenetic regulators [58] (**Figure 1**). These genetic alterations are often coincident with mutations in the prominent melanoma oncogenes *BRAF* and *NRAS*, suggesting that epigenetic reprogramming may modulate key oncogenic signaling pathways. Close inspection of the TCGA data also provides important clues to the functional relationships between various epigenetic regulators. For example, mutations in genes from related families, such as the histone methyltransferases *MLL* (*KMT2A*) and *MLL2* (*KMT2D*) or protein complexes, such as SWI/SNF, are often mutually exclusive (**Figure 1**). This suggests functional redundancies that may be important to melanoma biology. The data also reveals that a subset of melanomas harbor genomic amplifications that contain epigenetic genes, such as the histone methyltransferases *EZH2* and *SETDB1* (**Figure 1**). Overall, the high frequency of genetic alterations that impact chromatin regulators implicates epigenetic regulation as a driving force behind melanoma pathogenesis.

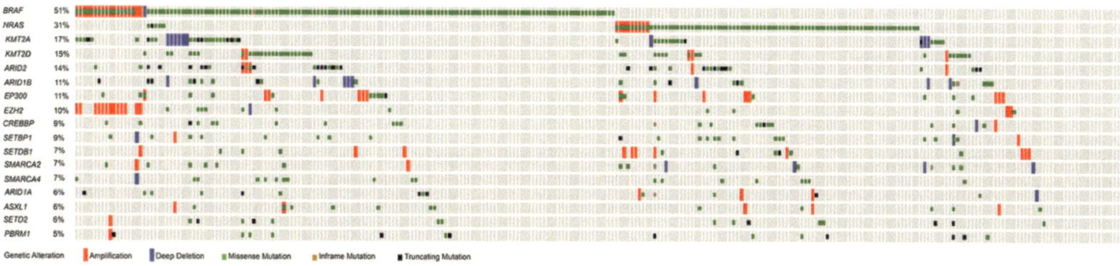

Figure 1. Prominent genetic alterations in epigenetic regulator genes in cutaneous melanoma. The oncogenes BRAF and NRAS are altered in 51% and 31% of the 278 melanoma tumor samples, respectively. Many of these tumors also harbor additional mutations in genes that encode for epigenetic factors. This figure highlights epigenetic genes that are altered in >5% of melanoma tumors. Data is publicly available courtesy of Memorial Sloan-Kettering Cancer Center's cBioPortal for Cancer Genomics (http://www.cbioportal.org).

5. Novel epigenetic drug targets in melanoma

The discovery of widespread epigenetic alterations in melanoma has led to the premise that melanoma patients would derive therapeutic benefit from therapies that reprogram cancer-specific gene expression patterns [25, 59]. To this end, first generation epigenetic therapies, such as DNA hypomethylating agents and histone deacetylase inhibitors, have made their way into melanoma clinical trials, primarily in combination with other therapeutic agents. Unfortunately, these early molecules lack selectivity and have demonstrated limited single-agent clinical activity outside of hematological malignancies, highlighting the need for therapies that target alternative epigenetic mechanisms and cellular pathways. The combination of genome-wide analyses and targeted genetic approaches has uncovered potential drug targets representing multiple classes of epigenetic regulators, including histone methyltransferases, histone demethylases, histone ubiquitin ligases, and epigenetic readers (**Table 1**). In addition, the prevalence of inactivating mutations in histone modifying enzymes and chromatin remodeling factors suggests the potential for identifying targetable vulnerabilities in the context of specific genetic backgrounds.

Target	Enzyme class	Therapeutic rationale in melanoma	References
EZH2	Histone Methyltransferase	Amplified and overexpressed gain-of-function mutations identified in 3% of patients. Genetic and pharmacological inhibition impairs tumor growth and metastasis	[53, 54, 70, 75, 77–79]
SETDB1	Histone Methyltransferase	Amplified and overexpressed. Accelerates tumor progression in zebrafish melanoma model	[86]
JARID1B	Histone Demethylase	Required for continuous tumor growth. Potential cancer stem cell marker. Potential role in mediating drug resistance	[96–98]
JMJD3	Histone Demethylase	Promotes growth and metastasis of melanoma cells. Modulates tumor microenvironment through NF-κB and BMP signaling	[105]
RNF2	Histone Ubiquitin Ligase	Overexpressed in melanoma. Part of gene signature that correlates with melanoma invasion. Dual role in tumor growth and invasion	[107–109]
BRD4	Bromodomain	Amplified and overexpressed. Genetic and pharmacological inhibition impairs tumor growth Potentiates Ras-driven transcription in *NF1*-mutant tumors	[119–123]

Table 1. Novel epigenetic drug targets in melanoma.

5.1. EZH2

Polycomb group (PcG) proteins are regulators of chromatin structure that play essential roles in transcriptional control during development [60, 61]. The histone methyltransferase EZH2 is the catalytic subunit of polycomb repressor complex 2 (PRC2), a conserved multiprotein complex that represses gene expression by methylating lysine 27 on histone H3 [62–64]. In the context of PRC2, EZH2 methyltransferase activity plays a key role in a number of biological processes, including cellular differentiation, X-inactivation, and stem cell pluripotency [65].

In addition to its normal roles in development, accumulating evidence supports an oncogenic role for EZH2 in the initiation and progression of a variety of cancers [66–68]. Overexpression of EZH2 has been observed in a wide range of tumor types, and elevated expression is often correlated with aggressive disease and poor prognosis [69, 70]. More recently, oncogenic gain-of-function mutations in EZH2 have been identified in DLBCL and FL that alter its enzymatic activity, resulting in elevated levels of H3K27me3 [56, 57]. Moreover, genetic and pharmacological inhibition of EZH2 enzymatic activity in both wild-type and mutant settings has been shown to inhibit cell proliferation and regress tumor growth, further validating EZH2 as a potential cancer target [71–73].

Several lines of evidence suggest that aberrant EZH2 activity plays a role in melanoma pathogenesis and progression. EZH2 expression has been shown to increase incrementally during the progression from benign nevi to malignant tumor [74]. To this end, EZH2 is genetically amplified in melanoma patient samples, and elevated expression has been shown to correlate with aggressive disease and poor survival [70, 75]. In addition, genetic depletion of EZH2 in human melanoma cells has been shown to inhibit cell proliferation *in vitro* and *in vivo* by inducing p21-/CDKN1A-mediated cellular senescence [76]. More recently, it was demonstrated that conditional ablation of *Ezh2* in a melanoma mouse model inhibited tumor growth and abolished metastasis without affecting normal melanocytes. Importantly, these effects were mimicked by pharmacological inhibition of EZH2 confirming the importance of EZH2 catalytic activity [77]. In addition to genetic amplification, whole-exome sequencing analysis has also identified previously characterized $EZH2^{Y641}$ gain-of-function mutations in melanoma tumors [54, 55]. While inhibition of EZH2 in melanoma cell lines harboring $EZH2^{Y641}$ mutations has been shown to inhibit cell proliferation and induce apoptosis, a study examining the growth of EZH2 mutant cells in three-dimensional assays also uncovered important roles in cell motility and migration that are independent of cell proliferation [78, 79]. The alterations in cell proliferation and motility are consistent with the proliferative and metastatic phenotypes reported following inhibition of wild-type EZH2 in mouse melanoma models [77]. Interestingly, $EZH2^{Y641}$ mutations appear to be coincident with $BRAF^{V600}$ mutations, suggesting an important link between epigenetic alterations and the MAPK pathway signaling [80]. This is supported by a recent finding that the combination of $Braf^{V600E}$ and $Ezh2^{Y641F}$ mutations accelerated disease progression in a melanoma mouse model [53].

5.2. SETDB1

SET domain bifurcated 1, or SETDB1, is a histone methyltransferase that mediates trimethylation of lysine 9 on histone H3 (H3K9me3) [81]. SETDB1 has been shown to be involved in the transcriptional silencing of both euchromatic genes and retro-elements [81–84]. The mechanism of transcriptional repression by SETDB1 may involve the DNA methylation machinery as SETDB1 was shown to be recruited to chromatin by the methyl-CpG-binding protein MBD1 to silence tumor suppressor genes, such as *RASSF1A* and *p53BP2* [83, 85]. In 2011, the *SETDB1* gene, located on chromosome band 1q21, was found to be amplified in several tumor types, including melanoma [86]. In the same study, expression of SETDB1 accelerated tumor progression in a zebrafish melanoma model harboring an oncogenic $BRAF^{V600E}$ mutation [86]. Chromatin immunoprecipitation coupled to gene expression analysis confirmed that increased levels of SETDB1 correlated with aberrant silencing of key genes involved in development [86].

On heels of the zebrafish study, there has been surprisingly little data in mammalian systems linking SETDB1 to melanoma progression. However, in addition to melanoma, SETDB1 is also focally amplified in non–small cell lung cancer, small cell cancer, ovarian cancer, hepatocellular carcinoma, prostate cancer, and breast cancer [86–91]. Emerging data in these settings suggests that elevated expression of SETDB1 may provide tumor cells with a growth advantage. For example, depletion of SETDB1 by siRNA or shRNA in *SETDB1*-amplified breast, liver, prostate, and lung cancer cells has been shown to inhibit proliferation *in vitro* and *in vivo*, indicating that these cells require elevated SETDB1 for their growth [87–89, 91]. In addition, inhibition of SETDB1 has been shown to negatively impact cell migration and invasion, suggesting that the role of SETDB1 may extend beyond the regulation of cell proliferation [88].

While the pathways that trigger cancer-specific overexpression of SETDB1 remain poorly elucidated, recent data has begun to shed light on the downstream mechanisms by which SETDB1 facilitates tumor growth in specific genetic contexts. SETDB1 has been shown to regulate the stability of tumor suppressors p53 and p53-related p63 [89, 91]. In 2015, Fei et al. reported the molecular interplay between SETDB1 and the well-known hotspot gain-of-function *TP53* R249S mutation. In this study, the authors demonstrated that SETDB1 catalyzes the demethylation of p53K370 and prevents the degradation of p53 by MDM2. More importantly, they found that inactivation of SETDB1 in HCC cell lines harboring R249S mutation suppresses cell growth, suggesting that *TP53* mutational status renders cancer cells dependent on SETDB1 activity. While reliance on the tumor suppressive capacity of p53 is profoundly emphasized by its near universal malfunction in all cancers and *TP53* is the most altered gene in cancer, accumulating evidence indicates that many mutant p53 isoforms can exert additional oncogenic activity by a gain-of-function mechanism [92–94]. With the recent observation that 19% of melanoma tumor harbor mutations in the *TP53* gene, the interplay between SETDB1 and p53 may suggest a therapeutic strategy for targeting melanoma patients with *TP53* mutations [54].

5.3. JARID1B

One of the main characteristics of melanoma is intratumor heterogeneity, as different subpopulations of cancer cells are found across patient samples. JARID1B (KDM5B) is a member of the highly conserved family of Jumonji proteins and is responsible for demethylation of methylated lysine 4 of histone H3 [95]. While highly expressed in benign nevi, JARID1B expression is restricted to ~5–10% of the total cell population in aggressive and metastatic melanomas [96]. Notably, even within highly proliferative melanomas, a JARID1B-positive subpopulation was present in a slow-cycling state [97]. Although not required for tumor initiation, elegant studies by Roesch et al. have demonstrated that JARID1B is required for the continuous tumor growth. While knockdown of JARID1B induces an initial burst of tumor growth, this is quickly exhausted [97]. Follow-on studies have shown that the JARID1B-positive subpopulation is intrinsically resistant to chemo- and targeted therapies [98]. While self-renewal and drug resistance are characteristics of stem-like cells, expression of JARID1B does not follow the classical hierarchical cancer stem cell model [97]. Overall, these studies provide valuable insight regarding the mechanisms of tumor heterogeneity and suggest the possibility of targeting JARID1B as a strategy for overcoming drug resistance in melanoma.

5.4. JMJD3

JMJD3 is a histone demethylase that is responsible for the removal of the trimethyl group from the H3K27 [99]. Several studies have shown that JMJD3 may play a dual role in human cancers, functioning as either a tumor suppressor or an oncogene depending on the cell type and cellular context [100–104]. Recently, an oncogenic role for JMJD3 was elucidated in melanoma [105]. Contrary to previous reports showing an antiproliferative effect of JMJD3 in different cancer types, JMJD3 promoted melanoma tumor growth and metastasis by modulating intrinsic cellular properties as well as the tumor microenvironment through PI3K signaling. Importantly, JMJD3 activity in melanoma cells was responsible for the transcriptional activation of target genes in the NF-κB and BMP signaling pathways [105]. Although additional work will need to be done to fully understand the mechanisms by which JMJD3-mediated modulation of H3K27 methylation promotes melanoma, this study provides the initial evidence linking epigenetic regulation by JMJD3 to melanoma progression and metastasis.

5.5. RNF2

Ubiquitination of histone tails is emerging as an important epigenetic modification in cancer. RNF2, an E3 ubiquitin ligase, is a core component of the polycomb repressive complex 1 (PRC1). In the context of PRC1, RNF2 promotes gene silencing by monoubiquitinating lysine 119 on histone H2A (H2AK119ub) [106]. RNF2 is overexpressed in multiple cancers and it is also part of an 18 gene signature that correlates with melanoma invasion [107]. Through a series of genetic studies in mouse and human systems, Rai et al. recently demonstrated that RNF2 plays a dual role in melanoma progression, regulating both tumorigenic and invasive potential [108]. Importantly, the proinvasive function of RNF2 was shown to require its E3 ligase activity, while its ability to promote tumor growth was independent of this catalytic function [108]. The TGF-β pathway is a key regulator of cancer cell invasion and metastasis. RNF2 potentiates TGF-β signaling by monoubiquitinating H2AK119 at the promoter of the LTBP2 gene, leading to the transcriptional repression of this negative regulator of the TGF-β pathway [108]. Given that the vast majority of melanoma deaths stem from metastatic disease, this mechanistic insight may provide an opportunity for future therapeutic intervention with catalytic inhibitors of RNF2. Interestingly, the noncatalytic function of RNF2 also provides important insight to potential therapies. MEK1-dependent phosphorylation of RNF2 leads to the formation of alternative complexes containing the histone demethylase KDM6A and the histone acetyltransferase EP300, which activate downstream target genes such as *CCND2* [108].This suggests the possibility of using RNF2 inhibitors in combination with either MEK or EP300 inhibitors to target both tumor growth and metastasis [109].

5.6. BRD4

In addition to the numerous chromatin modifying proteins and complexes, epigenetic readers also constitute key components of the mechanisms by which gene expression is regulated. First identified in members of the SWI/SNF and mediator complexes [110–112], bromodomains are found in many transcription factors and developmental regulators that control gene expression through histone modification and chromatin remodeling [113–115]. In addition to playing important roles in cell-cycle control during normal development, several bromodomain-containing proteins have also been implicated in cancer [116, 117]. The bromodomain and extraterminal (BET) protein family member BRD4 has gained considerable attention due to its aberrant activity in multiple cancer indications and its ability to drive expression of key oncogenes, such as *MYC* and *BCL2* [118]. BRD4 was found to be amplified or overexpressed in melanoma cell lines and primary tumors, and stable gene knockdown caused a significant reduction in tumor growth with significant impact on key cell-cycle genes [119]. In agreement with this genetic data, pharmacological inhibition of BRD4 has been shown to impair melanoma cell growth both *in vitro* and *in vivo*, further validating this epigenetic reader as a cancer target in this disease [119–121]. In addition, BET bromodomain inhibitors have been shown to selectively inhibit uveal melanoma cells harboring *Gnaq/11* mutations in a Myc-independent manner, suggesting a precision medicine strategy for therapeutic intervention [122]. Melanomas are also characterized by loss-of-function mutations in the gene encoding the Ras GTPase-activating protein *NF1* [123]. It was recently reported that the combined loss of *NF1* and the PRC2 component *SUZ12* amplifies RAS-driven transcription, and that this effect is mediated by BRD4 recruitment to H3K27Ac at downstream target genes [123]. This study also highlighted the therapeutic potential of simultaneously targeting BRD4 and the MAPK pathway.

5.7. Synthetic lethal strategies

SWI/SNF is evolutionarily conserved, ATP-dependent chromatin remodeling complex. Recent genome-wide sequencing approaches have revealed that subunits of SWI/SNF are recurrently mutated across many human cancers, including melanoma [32, 124, 125]. Although the roles of SWI/SNF complex in cancer are still poorly understood, studies indicate that SWI/SNF complexes may be master regulators of genes involved in cellular differentiation and that perturbations in the activity and stoichiometry of this complex promote tumorigenesis [126–128]. In melanoma, loss-of-function mutations have been identified in several genes encoding SWI/SNF components, including *ARID2, ARID1A, ARID1B, SMARCA2*, and *SMARCA4* [23, 54, 55]. Investigation into these deficiencies has begun to reveal tumor-specific referred dependencies that may represent druggable targets. For example, recent studies have identified putative synthetic lethal relationships in *SMARCA4*- and *ARID1A*-deficient tumors, where proliferation of the mutant cells depends on the activity of the closely related paralogs *SMARCA2* and *ARID1B* [129–132]. While similar dependencies have yet to be demonstrated in melanoma tumors harboring SWI/SNF mutations, these observations have at least opened up the possibility of treating melanoma patients with genetically defined mutations in the SWI/SNF complex. Recently, this concept of epigenetic synthetic lethality has been extended to *CBP/EP300*-deficient cancers [133]. EP300 and CBP are closely related chromatin modifying proteins facilitating acetylation of lysine residues on histones H3 and H4 [134, 135]. Genome-wide sequencing studies have revealed that multiple types of human cancers, including melanoma, harbor loss-of-function mutations in both *CBP* and *EP300* [136–139]. A recent study has identified EP300 as a key target in *CBP*-deficient cancer cells, describing another example of a paralog targeting strategy that specifically exploits human cancers harboring loss-of-function *CBP* mutations [133]. Given the frequency and mutually exclusive nature of *CBP* and *EP300* mutations in melanoma, the paralog targeting approach may provide an additional opportunity for targeting these epigenetically defined subsets of melanoma patients.

6. Clinical strategies for the treatment of melanoma with epigenetic inhibitors

6.1. First-generation epigenetic inhibitors: DNA hypomethylating agents and HDAC inhibitors

The initial foray into epigenetic therapy focused on the development of small molecule inhibitors to DNA methyltransferase (DNMT) and histone deacetylase enzymes, and these molecules are being explored as therapeutic modalities in multiple cancer types, including melanoma. However, treatment of solid tumors with these agents continues to be a challenge, with approvals in the clinic being limited to a subset of hematological malignancies [140]. In recent years, treatment paradigms have shifted toward the use of lower, transient doses that favor modulation of DNA and chromatin structure over general cytotoxicities [141]. Treatment strategies in melanoma are currently focused on drug combinations that override resistance mechanisms and potentiate antitumor immune responses (**Table 2**) [24].

Clinical trial name	Class of epigenetic therapy	Identifier	Phase
Study to Determine Efficacy and Safety of CC-486 with Nab-Paclitaxel in Patients with Chemotherapy Naïve Metastatic Melanoma	DNA Hypomethylating Agent	NCT01933061	II
Treatment of Resistant Disease Using Decitabine Combined with Vemurafenib Plus Cobimetinib	DNA Hypomethylating Agent	NCT01876641	I/II
Combination of Decitabine and Temozolomide in the Treatment of Patients with Metastatic Melanoma	DNA Hypomethylating Agent	NCT00715793	I/II
Parallel Trial of Decitabine and Peg-Interferon in Melanoma: Phase II Portion	DNA Hypomethylating Agent	NCT02605473	II
Parallel Trial of Decitabine and Peg-Interferon in Melanoma: Phase I Portion	DNA Hypomethylating Agent	NCT00791271	I
Azacitidine and Interferon Alfa in Treating Patients with Metastatic Melanoma	DNA Hypomethylating Agent	NCT00398450	I
Phase I/II Trial of Valproic Acid and Karenitecin for Melanoma	DNA Hypomethylating Agent	NCT00358319	I/II
Azacitidine and Recombinant Interferon Alfa-2B in Treating Patients with Stage III or IV Melanoma	DNA Hypomethylating Agent	NCT00217542	I
Decitabine in Treating Patients with Melanoma or Other Advanced Cancer	DNA Hypomethylating Agent	NCT00002980	I
Treatment of Resistant Metastatic Melanoma using	DNA Hypomethylating	NCT00925132	I/II

Clinical trial name	Class of epigenetic therapy	Identifier	Phase
Decitabine, Temozoomide and Panobinostat	Agent, HDAC inhibitor		
Ph1b/2 Dose Escalation Study of Entinostat with Pembrolizumab in NSCLC with Expansion Cohorts in NSCLC and Melanoma	HDAC Inhibitor	NCT02437136	I/II
Phase I of Histone Deacetylase Inhibitor Panobinostat with Ipilimumab with Unresectable II/IV melanoma	HDAC Inhibitor	NCT02032810	I
Vorinostat in Treating Patients with Metastatic Melanoma of the Eye	HDAC Inhibitor	NCT01587352	II
Proteasome inhibitor NPI-0052 and Vorinostat in Patients with NSCLC, pancreatic cancer, melanoma or lymphoma	HDAC Inhibitor	NCT00667082	I
Vorinostat in Treating Patients with Metastatic or Unresectable Melanoma	HDAC Inhibitor	NCT00121225	II
Safety and Efficacy of a New Chemotherapy Agent to Treat Metastatic Melanoma	HDAC Inhibitor	NCT00185302	II
MS-275 in Treating Patients with Advanced Solid Tumors or Lymphoma	HDAC Inhibitor	NCT00020579	I

Table 2. Melanoma clinical trials with epigenetic therapies.

6.1.1. Overcoming resistance to chemo- and targeted therapies

As stated earlier, rapid onset of drug resistance is a major impediment to targeted melanoma therapies. The observation that drug resistance is often accompanied by changes in chromatin structure and gene expression suggests the possibility of reversing this process through epigenetic therapy. To this end, increased expression of HDACs has been shown to mediate drug resistance in melanoma, and acquired resistance to vemurafenib in *BRAF*-mutant melanoma cells can be overcome when this agent is used in combination with HDAC inhibitors [142]. Epigenetic therapies are also being explored as a strategy for overcoming resistance to chemotherapy. For example, sequential treatment with the DNA hypomethylating agent decitabine and the HDAC inhibitor panobinostat is currently being explored in combination with temozolomide, a DNA alkylating agent, in metastatic melanoma (**Table 2**) [143]. Tumor necrosis factor-related apoptosis-inducing ligand (TRAIL) has shown promise in melanoma clinical trials; however, its utility has been limited by intrinsic and acquired resistance. The combination of TRAIL and the HDAC inhibitor entinostat was shown to override TRAIL resistance and induce cell death [144]. Resistance to interferon-based immunotherapy has been postulated to result from epigenetic silencing of interferon response genes. Treatment of melanoma cell lines with DNMT inhibitors has been shown to upregulate interferon response genes, such as *DR4* and *XAF1*, and augment the antiproliferative effects of interferon-alpha and interferon-beta [145, 146]. These examples highlight the potential use of epigenetic therapy to overcome resistance mechanisms that limit the efficacy of current melanoma therapies.

6.1.2. Combinations with immunotherapy

Durable survival benefits have been achieved in melanoma patients treated with immune checkpoint inhibitors [18–20]. Data in extensively treated patients with advanced non–small cell lung cancer suggests that this effect can be enhanced by combined epigenetic therapy. In this study, a subset of patients pretreated with a low-dose combination of the DNMT inhibitor 5-azacytidine and the HDAC inhibitor entinostat had major objective responses following subsequent treatment with immune checkpoint inhibitors [147]. Further mechanistic studies suggest that these agents may prime cancer cells to immunotherapy treatment by modulating immune response pathways [148, 149]. Intriguingly, this effect does not appear to be mediated through direct regulation of immune response genes, but rather by the upregulation of endogenous retroviruses that trigger viral immune response pathways [150, 151]. This observation has led to the hypothesis that epigenetic therapy activates innate immune response pathways by inducing a state of viral mimicry. In support of this premise, a retrospective analysis of RNA-seq data from melanoma patients treated with the immune checkpoint inhibitor anti-CTLA-4 revealed high levels of a viral defense signature in patients that correlated with long-term therapeutic benefit. Moreover, the authors went on to demonstrate that treatment with low-dose 5-azacytidine potentiates the antitumor activity of anti-CTLA-4 antibodies in a mouse melanoma model [150]. Epigenetic mechanisms also promote immune evasion by downregulating the expression of cell surface receptors and antigens required for immune recognition. Treatment of melanoma cell lines with DNMT and HDAC inhibitors induces the expression of tumor-associated antigens, costimulatory molecules, and MHC class I molecules, which unmask the tumor cell to allow T-cell-mediated responses [152–154]. In addition, epigenetic therapy has been shown to alter immunogenicity in melanoma cells by upregulating the expression of PD-L1, the ligand for the immune checkpoint molecule PD-1. In immunocompetent mice, the combination of HDAC inhibitor and PD-1 blockade inhibited tumor growth and significantly improved survival [155]. Taken together, these data highlight the potential for first-generation epigenetic drugs to augment the activity of immunotherapies in melanoma patients.

6.2. The emergence and promise of second-generation epigenetic therapies

The next generation of targeted epigenetic therapies has recently made its way into the clinic. In general, these agents are more selective than their first-generation counterparts and target a broader range of epigenetic mechanisms. Small molecule inhibitors of EZH2 are currently in phase I/II trials for the treatment of genetically defined tumors harboring mutations in *EZH2*, *INI1*, and *SMARCA4* [156]. The first of these agents, EPZ-6438, has demonstrated robust signs of clinical activity that extend beyond the original precision medicine hypothesis [157]. Preclinical data in both *EZH2* mutant and wild-type melanoma models demonstrating that EZH2 inhibitors negatively impact tumor growth and metastasis suggests that EZH2 inhibition will also be a promising strategy for treating melanoma patients [77, 79]. In addition to potential single agent studies, several lines of evidence support the pursuit of combination trials with current therapies. Recent studies in mice have uncovered a role for EZH2 in the maintenance of T regulatory (Treg) cell identity during cellular activation [158, 159]. In addition, EZH2 promotes immune evasion and suppression by directly repressing the expression of chemokines and cell surface antigens [75, 160, 161]. In both of these cases, EZH2 inhibition is likely to revert this immunosuppressive environment, rendering the tumor susceptible to immunotherapies. There is also the potential for using EZH2 inhibitors in combination with DNA methyltransferase inhibitors and/or HDAC inhibitors as these agents have demonstrated the ability to upregulate immune response pathways and synergize with immune checkpoint blockade therapy in non–small cell lung cancer [147, 148].

BET inhibitors modulate gene expression by disrupting the interaction between BET family bromodomains and acetylated lysine residues. Several BET inhibitors are currently being evaluated in the phase I/II clinical trials in multiple indications, and clinical proof of concept has recently been reported for OTX015/MK-8628 in patients with NUT midline carcinomas harboring the oncogenic BRD4-NUT translocation [162, 163]. This data highlights the potential for clinical application in additional indications. Treatment of melanoma cell lines with BET inhibitors leads to the rapid downregulation of cell-cycle genes and induces robust antiproliferative effects *in vitro* and *in vivo* [119, 120]. In addition, the combination of BET and HDAC inhibitors synergistically induces Bim-dependent apoptosis in melanoma cell lines and downregulates components of the AKT and YAP signaling pathways [164]. Most recently, important data has emerged around the role of BRD4 in drug resistance. In breast cancer cells that are intrinsically resistant to PI3K inhibitors, BRD4 participates in activation of upstream receptor tyrosine kinases to induce a feedback activation loop. The combination of the BET inhibitor JQ1 and the PI3K inhibitor GDC-0941 was able to overcome this resistance mechanism and inhibit tumor growth in multiple cancer models, suggesting a broad role for BRD4 in drug resistance [165]. Along these lines, it was also discovered that drug tolerant leukemia cells require BRD4 to maintain expression of proliferative and antiapoptotic genes, such as *MYC* and *BCL2* [166]. Treatment of this drug-resistant population with the BET inhibitor JQ1 resulted in downregulation of BRD4 target genes and induction of apoptosis. As stated earlier, the primary limitation of targeted therapies in melanoma is the rapid onset of acquired resistance. Given the emerging roles of BRD4 in this process, it is tempting to think that BET inhibitors could be used as a therapeutic strategy to overcome MAPK pathway-mediated drug resistance in melanoma patients. In addition, the ability of BET bromodomain inhibitors to modulate differentiation status and inflammatory functions of T cells warrants further investigation of their potential use in combination with targeted immunotherapies [167, 168].

While histone methyltransferase and BET bromodomain inhibitors continue to be evaluated in the clinic, there is increasing emphasis on the discovery of pharmacological inhibitors targeting other classes of epigenetic enzymes and chromatin regulators [169]. Catalytic inhibitors of the demethylases JMJD3 and JARID1B and the ubiquitin ligase RNF2 have been reported in the literature, and further optimization and preclinical evaluation in cancer models are underway [104, 170, 171]. In addition, potent inhibitors of bromodomains outside the well-characterized BET family have also recently been identified. These novel molecules are being pursued as alternative approaches to targeting epigenetic enzymes whose catalytic domains have been historically difficult to drug, such as the histone acetyltransferases and ATPase/helicases [172, 173]. The continued development of second-generation epigenetic therapies and the exploration of their use as single agents as well as in combination with targeted and immunotherapies is likely to have a significant impact on future treatment options for patients with advanced or metastatic melanoma.

7. Conclusions

It is becoming increasingly clear that epigenetic reprogramming is a hallmark of melanoma. In addition to changes in DNA methylation and histone acetylation, the advent of genome-wide whole-exome sequencing from patient samples has revealed a high incidence of genetic alterations in genes from key families of epigenetic regulators. The identification of gene amplifications and activating mutations, in addition to gene deletions and inactivating mutations, indicates that an individual epigenetic regulator may play either an oncogenic or tumor suppressive role depending on the genetic background or stage of the disease. Importantly, further interrogation in human and mouse cancer models has led to the identification of several proteins that appear to play important roles in melanoma growth, metastasis, and stem cell renewal, suggesting that they may be bona fide cancer targets. DNA hypomethylating agents and histone deacetylase inhibitors, the first generation of epigenetic therapies, continue to be evaluated in clinical trials, primarily in combination with chemo-, targeted, and immunotherapies. The second generation of epigenetic inhibitors are highly selective and target novel epigenetic mechanisms that regulate multiple facets of cancer biology, including cell proliferation, cell migration, metastasis, stem cell renewal, drug resistance, and immune regulation. While it remains to be seen if these epigenetic targets are oncogenic drivers in the strict sense, they may cooperate with other oncogenes (for example, *BRAF*) to fine tune the transcriptional landscape in melanoma cells to promote tumorigenesis, confer drug resistance and evade immune responses. As they continue to make their way into the clinic, this next generation of novel epigenetic therapies will provide opportunities for multiple levels of therapeutic intervention for melanoma patients. Moreover, further exploration of the evolving melanoma landscape will continue to uncover novel epigenetic mechanisms and guide the future generations of epigenetic therapy.

Author details

Robert A. Rollins*, Kimberly H. Kim and Cheng-Chung Tsao

*Address all correspondence to: robert.rollins@pfizer.com

Pfizer, Inc, Oncology Research & Development, Pearl River, New York, USA

References

[1] AIM at Melanoma Foundation. "Melanoma Stats, Facts, and Figures". Plano: AIM at Melanoma Foundation; 2016.

[2] American Cancer Society. "Cancer Facts and Figures 2016". Atlanta: American Cancer Society; 2016.

[3] Chin L. The genetics of malignant melanoma: lessons from mouse and man. Nature Reviews Cancer. 2003;3(8):559–570.

[4] Mort RL, Jackson IJ, Patton EE. The melanocyte lineage in development and disease. Development. 2015;142(4):620–632.

[5] Karachaliou N, Pilotto S, Teixido C, Viteri S, Gonzalez-Cao M, Riso A, et al. Melanoma: oncogenic drivers and the immune system. Annals of Translational Medicine. 2015;3(18):265.

[6] Dhomen N, Marais R. BRAF signaling and targeted therapies in melanoma. Hematology/Oncology Clinics of North America. 2009;23(3):529–545, ix.

[7] Milagre C, Dhomen N, Geyer FC, Hayward R, Lambros M, Reis-Filho JS, et al. A mouse model of melanoma driven by oncogenic KRAS. Cancer Research. 2010;70(13):5549–5557.

[8] Bollag G, Hirth P, Tsai J, Zhang J, Ibrahim PN, Cho H, et al. Clinical efficacy of a RAF inhibitor needs broad target blockade in BRAF-mutant melanoma. Nature. 2010;467(7315):596–599.

[9] Flaherty KT, Puzanov I, Kim KB, Ribas A, McArthur GA, Sosman JA, et al. Inhibition of mutated, activated BRAF in metastatic melanoma. The New England Journal of Medicine. 2010;363(9):809–819.

[10] Chapman PB, Hauschild A, Robert C, Haanen JB, Ascierto P, Larkin J, et al. Improved survival with vemurafenib in melanoma with BRAF V600E mutation. The New England Journal of Medicine. 2011;364(26):2507–2516.

[11] Flaherty KT, Robert C, Hersey P, Nathan P, Garbe C, Milhem M, et al. Improved survival with MEK inhibition in BRAF-mutated melanoma. The New England Journal of Medicine. 2012;367(2):107–114.

[12] Hauschild A, Grob JJ, Demidov LV, Jouary T, Gutzmer R, Millward M, et al. Dabrafenib in BRAF-mutated metastatic melanoma: a multicentre, open-label, phase 3 randomised controlled trial. Lancet. 2012;380(9839):358–365.

[13] Nazarian R, Shi H, Wang Q, Kong X, Koya RC, Lee H, et al. Melanomas acquire resistance to B-RAF(V600E) inhibition by RTK or N-RAS upregulation. Nature. 2010;468(7326):973–977.

[14] Oberholzer PA, Kee D, Dziunycz P, Sucker A, Kamsukom N, Jones R, et al. RAS mutations are associated with the development of cutaneous squamous cell tumors in patients treated with RAF inhibitors. Journal of Clinical Oncology. 2012;30(3):316–321.

[15] Flaherty KT, Infante JR, Daud A, Gonzalez R, Kefford RF, Sosman J, et al. Combined BRAF and MEK inhibition in melanoma with BRAF V600 mutations. The New England Journal of Medicine. 2012;367(18):1694–1703.

[16] Long GV, Stroyakovskiy D, Gogas H, Levchenko E, de Braud F, Larkin J, et al. Combined BRAF and MEK inhibition versus BRAF inhibition alone in melanoma. The New England Journal of Medicine. 2014;371(20):1877–1888.

[17] Moriceau G, Hugo W, Hong A, Shi H, Kong X, Yu CC, et al. Tunable-combinatorial mechanisms of acquired resistance limit the efficacy of BRAF/MEK cotargeting but result in melanoma drug addiction. Cancer Cell. 2015;27(2):240–256.

[18] Robert C, Schachter J, Long GV, Arance A, Grob JJ, Mortier L, et al. Pembrolizumab versus Ipilimumab in Advanced Melanoma. The New England Journal of Medicine. 2015;372(26):2521–2532.

[19] Topalian SL, Hodi FS, Brahmer JR, Gettinger SN, Smith DC, McDermott DF, et al. Safety, activity, and immune correlates of anti-PD-1 antibody in cancer. The New England Journal of Medicine. 2012;366(26):2443–2454.

[20] Hodi FS, O'Day SJ, McDermott DF, Weber RW, Sosman JA, Haanen JB, et al. Improved survival with ipilimumab in patients with metastatic melanoma. The New England Journal of Medicine. 2010;363(8):711–723.

[21] Ribas A, Hodi FS, Callahan M, Konto C, Wolchok J. Hepatotoxicity with combination of vemurafenib and ipilimumab. The New England Journal of Medicine. 2013;368(14): 1365–1366.

[22] Hu-Lieskovan S, Robert L, Homet Moreno B, Ribas A. Combining targeted therapy with immunotherapy in BRAF-mutant melanoma: promise and challenges. Journal of Clinical Oncology. 2014;32(21):2248–2254.

[23] Lee JJ, Sholl LM, Lindeman NI, Granter SR, Laga AC, Shivdasani P, et al. Targeted next-generation sequencing reveals high frequency of mutations in epigenetic regulators across treatment-naive patient melanomas. Clinical Epigenetics. 2015;7(1):59.

[24] Gallagher SJ, Tiffen JC, Hersey P. Histone modifications, modifiers and readers in melanoma resistance to targeted and immune therapy. Cancers. 2015;7(4):1959–1982.

[25] Sarkar D, Leung EY, Baguley BC, Finlay GJ, Askarian-Amiri ME. Epigenetic regulation in human melanoma: past and future. Epigenetics. 2015;10(2):103–121.

[26] Holliday R. DNA methylation and epigenetic mechanisms. Cell Biophysics. 1989;15(1–2):15–20.

[27] Simo-Riudalbas L, Esteller M. Targeting the histone orthography of cancer: drugs for writers, erasers and readers. British Journal of Pharmacology. 2015;172(11):2716–2732.

[28] Musselman CA, Lalonde ME, Cote J, Kutateladze TG. Perceiving the epigenetic landscape through histone readers. Nature Structural & Molecular Biology. 2012;19(12): 1218–1227.

[29] Azad N, Zahnow CA, Rudin CM, Baylin SB. The future of epigenetic therapy in solid tumours--lessons from the past. Nature Reviews Clinical Oncology. 2013;10(5):256–266.

[30] Garraway LA, Lander ES. Lessons from the cancer genome. Cell. 2013;153(1):17–37.

[31] Kandoth C, McLellan MD, Vandin F, Ye K, Niu B, Lu C, et al. Mutational landscape and significance across 12 major cancer types. Nature. 2013;502(7471):333–339.

[32] Kadoch C, Hargreaves DC, Hodges C, Elias L, Ho L, Ranish J, et al. Proteomic and bioinformatic analysis of mammalian SWI/SNF complexes identifies extensive roles in human malignancy. Nature Genetics. 2013;45(6):592–601.

[33] Rivera CM, Ren B. Mapping human epigenomes. Cell. 2013;155(1):39–55.

[34] Roadmap Epigenomics C, Kundaje A, Meuleman W, Ernst J, Bilenky M, Yen A, et al. Integrative analysis of 111 reference human epigenomes. Nature. 2015;518(7539):317–330.

[35] Berdasco M, Esteller M. Aberrant epigenetic landscape in cancer: how cellular identity goes awry. Developmental Cell. 2010;19(5):698–711.

[36] Esteller M. CpG island hypermethylation and tumor suppressor genes: a booming present, a brighter future. Oncogene. 2002;21(35):5427–5440.

[37] Esteller M, Herman JG. Cancer as an epigenetic disease: DNA methylation and chromatin alterations in human tumours. The Journal of Pathology. 2002;196(1):1–7.

[38] Ehrlich M. DNA hypomethylation in cancer cells. Epigenomics. 2009;1(2):239–259.

[39] Besaratinia A, Tommasi S. Epigenetics of human melanoma: promises and challenges. Journal of Molecular Cell Biology. 2014;6(5):356–367.

[40] Schinke C, Mo Y, Yu Y, Amiri K, Sosman J, Greally J, et al. Aberrant DNA methylation in malignant melanoma. Melanoma Research. 2010;20(4):253–265.

[41] Tanemura A, Terando AM, Sim MS, van Hoesel AQ, de Maat MF, Morton DL, et al. CpG island methylator phenotype predicts progression of malignant melanoma. Clinical Cancer Research. 2009;15(5):1801–1807.

[42] Sigalotti L, Fratta E, Bidoli E, Covre A, Parisi G, Colizzi F, et al. Methylation levels of the "long interspersed nucleotide element-1" repetitive sequences predict survival of melanoma patients. Journal of Translational Medicine. 2011;9:78.

[43] Guo X, Xu Y, Zhao Z. In-depth genomic data analyses revealed complex transcriptional and epigenetic dysregulations of BRAFV600E in melanoma. Molecular Cancer. 2015;14:60.

[44] Fang M, Hutchinson L, Deng A, Green MR. Common BRAF(V600E)-directed pathway mediates widespread epigenetic silencing in colorectal cancer and melanoma. Proceedings of the National Academy of Sciences of the United States of America. 2016;113(5):1250–1255.

[45] Sigalotti L, Covre A, Fratta E, Parisi G, Sonego P, Colizzi F, et al. Whole genome methylation profiles as independent markers of survival in stage IIIC melanoma patients. Journal of Translational Medicine. 2012;10:185.

[46] Lauss M, Ringner M, Karlsson A, Harbst K, Busch C, Geisler J, et al. DNA methylation subgroups in melanoma are associated with proliferative and immunological processes. BMC Medical Genomics. 2015;8:73.

[47] Venza M, Visalli M, Biondo C, Lentini M, Catalano T, Teti D, et al. Epigenetic regulation of p14ARF and p16INK4A expression in cutaneous and uveal melanoma. Biochimica et Biophysica Acta. 2015;1849(3):247–256.

[48] Liu J, Gu J, Feng Z, Yang Y, Zhu N, Lu W, et al. Both HDAC5 and HDAC6 are required for the proliferation and metastasis of melanoma cells. Journal of Translational Medicine. 2016;14:7.

[49] Jin SG, Xiong W, Wu X, Yang L, Pfeifer GP. The DNA methylation landscape of human melanoma. Genomics. 2015;106(6):322–330.

[50] Sengupta D, Byrum SD, Avaritt NL, Davis L, Shields B, Mahmoud F, et al. Quantitative histone mass spectrometry identifies elevated histone H3 lysine 27 (Lys27) trimethylation in melanoma. Molecular & Cellular Proteomics. 2016;15(3):765–775.

[51] Kampilafkos P, Melachrinou M, Kefalopoulou Z, Lakoumentas J, Sotiropoulou-Bonikou G. Epigenetic modifications in cutaneous malignant melanoma: EZH2, H3K4me2, and H3K27me3 immunohistochemical expression is enhanced at the invasion front of the tumor. The American Journal of Dermatopathology. 2015;37(2):138–144.

[52] Verfaillie A, Imrichova H, Atak ZK, Dewaele M, Rambow F, Hulselmans G, et al. Decoding the regulatory landscape of melanoma reveals TEADS as regulators of the invasive cell state. Nature Communications. 2015;6:6683.

[53] Souroullas GP, Jeck WR, Parker JS, Simon JM, Liu JY, Paulk J, et al. An oncogenic Ezh2 mutation induces tumors through global redistribution of histone 3 lysine 27 trimethylation. Nature Medicine 2016;22(6):632–640.

[54] Hodis E, Watson IR, Kryukov GV, Arold ST, Imielinski M, Theurillat JP, et al. A landscape of driver mutations in melanoma. Cell. 2012;150(2):251–263.

[55] Krauthammer M, Kong Y, Ha BH, Evans P, Bacchiocchi A, McCusker JP, et al. Exome sequencing identifies recurrent somatic RAC1 mutations in melanoma. Nature Genetics. 2012;44(9):1006–1014.

[56] Sneeringer CJ, Scott MP, Kuntz KW, Knutson SK, Pollock RM, Richon VM, et al. Coordinated activities of wild-type plus mutant EZH2 drive tumor-associated hyper-trimethylation of lysine 27 on histone H3 (H3K27) in human B-cell lymphomas. Proceedings of the National Academy of Sciences of the United States of America. 2010;107(49):20980–20985.

[57] Yap DB, Chu J, Berg T, Schapira M, Cheng SW, Moradian A, et al. Somatic mutations at EZH2 Y641 act dominantly through a mechanism of selectively altered PRC2 catalytic activity, to increase H3K27 trimethylation. Blood. 2011;117(8):2451–2459.

[58] Cancer Genome Atlas N. Genomic Classification of Cutaneous Melanoma. Cell. 2015;161(7):1681–1696.

[59] Lee JJ, Murphy GF, Lian CG. Melanoma epigenetics: novel mechanisms, markers, and medicines. Laboratory investigation. 2014;94(8):822–838.

[60] Sparmann A, van Lohuizen M. Polycomb silencers control cell fate, development and cancer. Nature Reviews Cancer. 2006;6(11):846–856.

[61] Bracken AP, Helin K. Polycomb group proteins: navigators of lineage pathways led astray in cancer. Nature Reviews Cancer. 2009;9(11):773–784.

[62] Czermin B, Melfi R, McCabe D, Seitz V, Imhof A, Pirrotta V. Drosophila enhancer of Zeste/ESC complexes have a histone H3 methyltransferase activity that marks chromosomal Polycomb sites. Cell. 2002;111(2):185–196.

[63] Cao R, Wang L, Wang H, Xia L, Erdjument-Bromage H, Tempst P, et al. Role of histone H3 lysine 27 methylation in Polycomb-group silencing. Science. 2002;298(5595):1039–1043.

[64] Muller J, Hart CM, Francis NJ, Vargas ML, Sengupta A, Wild B, et al. Histone methyltransferase activity of a Drosophila Polycomb group repressor complex. Cell. 2002;111(2):197–208.

[65] Cao R, Zhang Y. The functions of E(Z)/EZH2-mediated methylation of lysine 27 in histone H3. Current Opinion in Genetics & Development. 2004;14(2):155–164.

[66] Chase A, Cross NC. Aberrations of EZH2 in cancer. Clinical Cancer Research. 2011;17(9):2613–2618.

[67] Chang CJ, Hung MC. The role of EZH2 in tumour progression. British Journal of Cancer. 2012;106(2):243–247.

[68] McCabe MT, Creasy CL. EZH2 as a potential target in cancer therapy. Epigenomics. 2014;6(3):341–351.

[69] Kleer CG, Cao Q, Varambally S, Shen R, Ota I, Tomlins SA, et al. EZH2 is a marker of aggressive breast cancer and promotes neoplastic transformation of breast epithelial cells. Proceedings of the National Academy of Sciences of the United States of America. 2003;100(20):11606–11611.

[70] Bachmann IM, Halvorsen OJ, Collett K, Stefansson IM, Straume O, Haukaas SA, et al. EZH2 expression is associated with high proliferation rate and aggressive tumor subgroups in cutaneous melanoma and cancers of the endometrium, prostate, and breast. Journal of Clinical Oncology. 2006;24(2):268–273.

[71] Varambally S, Dhanasekaran SM, Zhou M, Barrette TR, Kumar-Sinha C, Sanda MG, et al. The polycomb group protein EZH2 is involved in progression of prostate cancer. Nature. 2002;419(6907):624–629.

[72] McCabe MT, Ott HM, Ganji G, Korenchuk S, Thompson C, Van Aller GS, et al. EZH2 inhibition as a therapeutic strategy for lymphoma with EZH2-activating mutations. Nature. 2012;492(7427):108–112.

[73] Knutson SK, Kawano S, Minoshima Y, Warholic NM, Huang KC, Xiao Y, et al. Selective inhibition of EZH2 by EPZ-6438 leads to potent antitumor activity in EZH2-mutant non-Hodgkin lymphoma. Molecular Cancer Therapeutics. 2014;13(4):842–854.

[74] McHugh JB, Fullen DR, Ma L, Kleer CG, Su LD. Expression of polycomb group protein EZH2 in nevi and melanoma. Journal of Cutaneous Pathology. 2007;34(8):597–600.

[75] Tiffen J, Wilson S, Gallagher SJ, Hersey P, Filipp FV. Somatic copy number amplification and hyperactivating somatic mutations of EZH2 correlate with DNA methylation and drive epigenetic silencing of genes involved in tumor suppression and immune responses in melanoma. Neoplasia. 2016;18(2):121–132.

[76] Fan T, Jiang S, Chung N, Alikhan A, Ni C, Lee CC, et al. EZH2-dependent suppression of a cellular senescence phenotype in melanoma cells by inhibition of p21/CDKN1A expression. Molecular Cancer Research. 2011;9(4):418–429.

[77] Zingg D, Debbache J, Schaefer SM, Tuncer E, Frommel SC, Cheng P, et al. The epigenetic modifier EZH2 controls melanoma growth and metastasis through silencing of distinct tumour suppressors. Nature Communications. 2015;6:6051.

[78] Barsotti AM, Ryskin M, Zhong W, Zhang WG, Giannakou A, Loreth C, et al. Epigenetic reprogramming by tumor-derived EZH2 gain-of-function mutations promotes aggressive 3D cell morphologies and enhances melanoma tumor growth. Oncotarget. 2015;6(5):2928–2938.

[79] Tiffen JC, Gunatilake D, Gallagher SJ, Gowrishankar K, Heinemann A, Cullinane C, et al. Targeting activating mutations of EZH2 leads to potent cell growth inhibition in human melanoma by derepression of tumor suppressor genes. Oncotarget. 2015;6(29): 27023–27036.

[80] Harms PW, Collie AM, Hovelson DH, Cani AK, Verhaegen ME, Patel RM, et al. Next generation sequencing of Cytokeratin 20-negative Merkel cell carcinoma reveals

ultraviolet-signature mutations and recurrent TP53 and RB1 inactivation. Modern Pathology. 2016;29(3):240–248.

[81] Schultz DC, Ayyanathan K, Negorev D, Maul GG, Rauscher FJ, 3rd. SETDB1: a novel KAP-1-associated histone H3, lysine 9-specific methyltransferase that contributes to HP1-mediated silencing of euchromatic genes by KRAB zinc-finger proteins. Genes & Development. 2002;16(8):919–932.

[82] Yang L, Xia L, Wu DY, Wang H, Chansky HA, Schubach WH, et al. Molecular cloning of ESET, a novel histone H3-specific methyltransferase that interacts with ERG transcription factor. Oncogene. 2002;21(1):148–152.

[83] Hunter C, Smith R, Cahill DP, Stephens P, Stevens C, Teague J, et al. A hypermutation phenotype and somatic MSH6 mutations in recurrent human malignant gliomas after alkylator chemotherapy. Cancer Research. 2006;66(8):3987–3991.

[84] Karimi MM, Goyal P, Maksakova IA, Bilenky M, Leung D, Tang JX, et al. DNA methylation and SETDB1/H3K9me3 regulate predominantly distinct sets of genes, retroelements, and chimeric transcripts in mESCs. Cell Stem Cell. 2011;8(6):676–687.

[85] Parry L, Clarke AR. The roles of the methyl-CpG binding proteins in cancer. Genes & Cancer. 2011;2(6):618–630.

[86] Ceol CJ, Houvras Y, Jane-Valbuena J, Bilodeau S, Orlando DA, Battisti V, et al. The histone methyltransferase SETDB1 is recurrently amplified in melanoma and accelerates its onset. Nature. 2011;471(7339):513–517.

[87] Rodriguez-Paredes M, Martinez de Paz A, Simo-Riudalbas L, Sayols S, Moutinho C, Moran S, et al. Gene amplification of the histone methyltransferase SETDB1 contributes to human lung tumorigenesis. Oncogene. 2014;33(21):2807–2813.

[88] Sun Y, Wei M, Ren SC, Chen R, Xu WD, Wang FB, et al. Histone methyltransferase SETDB1 is required for prostate cancer cell proliferation, migration and invasion. Asian Journal of Andrology. 2014;16(2):319–324.

[89] Regina C, Compagnone M, Peschiaroli A, Lena A, Annicchiarico-Petruzzelli M, Piro MC, et al. Setdb1, a novel interactor of DeltaNp63, is involved in breast tumorigenesis. Oncotarget 2016;7(20):28836–28848.

[90] Liu L, Kimball S, Liu H, Holowatyj A, Yang ZQ. Genetic alterations of histone lysine methyltransferases and their significance in breast cancer. Oncotarget. 2015;6(4):2466–2482.

[91] Fei Q, Shang K, Zhang J, Chuai S, Kong D, Zhou T, et al. Histone methyltransferase SETDB1 regulates liver cancer cell growth through methylation of p53. Nature Communications. 2015;6:8651.

[92] Zhou G, Wang J, Zhao M, Xie TX, Tanaka N, Sano D, et al. Gain-of-function mutant p53 promotes cell growth and cancer cell metabolism via inhibition of AMPK activation. Molecular Cell. 2014;54(6):960–974.

[93] Zhu J, Sammons MA, Donahue G, Dou Z, Vedadi M, Getlik M, et al. Gain-of-function p53 mutants co-opt chromatin pathways to drive cancer growth. Nature. 2015;525(7568):206–211.

[94] Ali A, Shah AS, Ahmad A. Gain-of-function of mutant p53: mutant p53 enhances cancer progression by inhibiting KLF17 expression in invasive breast carcinoma cells. Cancer Letters. 2014;354(1):87–96.

[95] Blair LP, Cao J, Zou MR, Sayegh J, Yan Q. Epigenetic regulation by lysine demethylase 5 (KDM5) enzymes in cancer. Cancers. 2011;3(1):1383–1404.

[96] Roesch A, Becker B, Meyer S, Wild P, Hafner C, Landthaler M, et al. Retinoblastoma-binding protein 2-homolog 1: a retinoblastoma-binding protein downregulated in malignant melanomas. Modern Pathology. 2005;18(9):1249–1257.

[97] Roesch A, Fukunaga-Kalabis M, Schmidt EC, Zabierowski SE, Brafford PA, Vultur A, et al. A temporarily distinct subpopulation of slow-cycling melanoma cells is required for continuous tumor growth. Cell. 2010;141(4):583–594.

[98] Roesch A, Vultur A, Bogeski I, Wang H, Zimmermann KM, Speicher D, et al. Overcoming intrinsic multidrug resistance in melanoma by blocking the mitochondrial respiratory chain of slow-cycling JARID1B(high) cells. Cancer Cell. 2013;23(6):811–825.

[99] Xiang Y, Zhu Z, Han G, Lin H, Xu L, Chen CD. JMJD3 is a histone H3K27 demethylase. Cell Research. 2007;17(10):850–857.

[100] Svotelis A, Bianco S, Madore J, Huppe G, Nordell-Markovits A, Mes-Masson AM, et al. H3K27 demethylation by JMJD3 at a poised enhancer of anti-apoptotic gene BCL2 determines ERalpha ligand dependency. The EMBO Journal. 2011;30(19):3947–3961.

[101] Agger K, Cloos PA, Rudkjaer L, Williams K, Andersen G, Christensen J, et al. The H3K27me3 demethylase JMJD3 contributes to the activation of the INK4A-ARF locus in response to oncogene- and stress-induced senescence. Genes & Development. 2009;23(10):1171–1176.

[102] Barradas M, Anderton E, Acosta JC, Li S, Banito A, Rodriguez-Niedenfuhr M, et al. Histone demethylase JMJD3 contributes to epigenetic control of INK4a/ARF by oncogenic RAS. Genes & Development. 2009;23(10):1177–1182.

[103] Ene CI, Edwards L, Riddick G, Baysan M, Woolard K, Kotliarova S, et al. Histone demethylase Jumonji D3 (JMJD3) as a tumor suppressor by regulating p53 protein nuclear stabilization. PloS One. 2012;7(12):e51407.

[104] Ntziachristos P, Tsirigos A, Welstead GG, Trimarchi T, Bakogianni S, Xu L, et al. Contrasting roles of histone 3 lysine 27 demethylases in acute lymphoblastic leukaemia. Nature. 2014;514(7523):513–517.

[105] Park WY, Hong BJ, Lee J, Choi C, Kim MY. H3K27 Demethylase JMJD3 employs the NF-kappaB and BMP signaling pathways to modulate the tumor microenvironment and promote melanoma progression and metastasis. Cancer Research. 2016;76(1):161–170.

[106] Di Croce L, Helin K. Transcriptional regulation by Polycomb group proteins. Nature Structural & Molecular Biology. 2013;20(10):1147–1155.

[107] Scott KL, Nogueira C, Heffernan TP, van Doorn R, Dhakal S, Hanna JA, et al. Proinvasion metastasis drivers in early-stage melanoma are oncogenes. Cancer Cell. 2011;20(1): 92–103.

[108] Rai K, Akdemir KC, Kwong LN, Fiziev P, Wu CJ, Keung EZ, et al. Dual Roles of RNF2 in Melanoma Progression. Cancer Discovery. 2015;5(12):1314–1327.

[109] Black JC, Whetstine JR. RNF2 E3 or not to E3: dual roles of RNF2 overexpression in melanoma. Cancer Discovery. 2015;5(12):1241–1243.

[110] Jiang YW, Veschambre P, Erdjument-Bromage H, Tempst P, Conaway JW, Conaway RC, et al. Mammalian mediator of transcriptional regulation and its possible role as an endpoint of signal transduction pathways. Proceedings of the National Academy of Sciences United States of America. 1998;95(15):8538–8543.

[111] Kuras L, Borggrefe T, Kornberg RD. Association of the Mediator complex with enhancers of active genes. Proceedings of the National Academy of Sciences of the United States of America. 2003;100(24):13887–13891.

[112] Dhalluin C, Carlson JE, Zeng L, He C, Aggarwal AK, Zhou MM. Structure and ligand of a histone acetyltransferase bromodomain. Nature. 1999;399(6735): 491–496.

[113] Haynes SR, Dollard C, Winston F, Beck S, Trowsdale J, Dawid IB. The bromodomain: a conserved sequence found in human, Drosophila and yeast proteins. Nucleic Acids Research. 1992;20(10):2603.

[114] Jeanmougin F, Wurtz JM, Le Douarin B, Chambon P, Losson R. The bromodomain revisited. Trends in Biochemical Sciences. 1997;22(5):151–153.

[115] Winston F, Allis CD. The bromodomain: a chromatin-targeting module? Nature Structural & Molecular Biology. 1999;6(7):601–604.

[116] Maruyama T, Farina A, Dey A, Cheong J, Bermudez VP, Tamura T, et al. A Mammalian bromodomain protein, brd4, interacts with replication factor C and inhibits progression to S phase. Molecular and Cellular Biology. 2002;22(18):6509–6520.

[117] Dey A, Chitsaz F, Abbasi A, Misteli T, Ozato K. The double bromodomain protein Brd4 binds to acetylated chromatin during interphase and mitosis. Proceedings of the National Academy of Sciences of the United States of America. 2003;100(15):8758–8763.

[118] Wyce A, Ganji G, Smitheman KN, Chung CW, Korenchuk S, Bai Y, et al. BET inhibition silences expression of MYCN and BCL2 and induces cytotoxicity in neuroblastoma tumor models. PloS One. 2013;8(8):e72967.

[119] Segura MF, Fontanals-Cirera B, Gaziel-Sovran A, Guijarro MV, Hanniford D, Zhang G, et al. BRD4 sustains melanoma proliferation and represents a new target for epigenetic therapy. Cancer Research. 2013;73(20):6264–6276.

[120] Gallagher SJ, Mijatov B, Gunatilake D, Tiffen JC, Gowrishankar K, Jin L, et al. The epigenetic regulator I-BET151 induces BIM-dependent apoptosis and cell cycle arrest of human melanoma cells. The Journal of Investigative Dermatology. 2014;134(11): 2795–2805.

[121] Conery AR, Centore RC, Spillane KL, Follmer NE, Bommi-Reddy A, Hatton C, et al. Preclinical anticancer efficacy of BET Bromodomain inhibitors is determined by the apoptotic response. Cancer Research. 2016;76(6):1313–1319.

[122] Ambrosini G, Sawle AD, Musi E, Schwartz GK. BRD4-targeted therapy induces Myc-independent cytotoxicity in Gnaq/11-mutatant uveal melanoma cells. Oncotarget. 2015;6(32):33397–33409.

[123] De Raedt T, Beert E, Pasmant E, Luscan A, Brems H, Ortonne N, et al. PRC2 loss amplifies Ras-driven transcription and confers sensitivity to BRD4-based therapies. Nature. 2014;514(7521):247–251.

[124] Masliah-Planchon J, Bieche I, Guinebretiere JM, Bourdeaut F, Delattre O. SWI/SNF chromatin remodeling and human malignancies. Annual Review of Pathology. 2015;10:145–171.

[125] Shain AH, Pollack JR. The spectrum of SWI/SNF mutations, ubiquitous in human cancers. PloS One. 2013;8(1):e55119.

[126] Keenen B, Qi H, Saladi SV, Yeung M, de la Serna IL. Heterogeneous SWI/SNF chromatin remodeling complexes promote expression of microphthalmia-associated transcription factor target genes in melanoma. Oncogene. 2010;29(1):81–92.

[127] Lin H, Wong RP, Martinka M, Li G. BRG1 expression is increased in human cutaneous melanoma. The British Journal of Dermatology. 2010;163(3):502–510.

[128] Vinod Saladi S, Marathe H, de la Serna IL. SWItching on the transcriptional circuitry in melanoma. Epigenetics. 2010;5(6):469–475.

[129] Hoffman GR, Rahal R, Buxton F, Xiang K, McAllister G, Frias E, et al. Functional epigenetics approach identifies BRM/SMARCA2 as a critical synthetic lethal target in

BRG1-deficient cancers. Proceedings of the National Academy of Sciences of the United States of America. 2014;111(8):3128–3133.

[130] Wilson BG, Helming KC, Wang X, Kim Y, Vazquez F, Jagani Z, et al. Residual complexes containing SMARCA2 (BRM) underlie the oncogenic drive of SMARCA4 (BRG1) mutation. Molecular and Cellular Biology. 2014;34(6):1136–1144.

[131] Oike T, Ogiwara H, Tominaga Y, Ito K, Ando O, Tsuta K, et al. A synthetic lethality-based strategy to treat cancers harboring a genetic deficiency in the chromatin remodeling factor BRG1. Cancer Research. 2013;73(17):5508–5518.

[132] Helming KC, Wang X, Wilson BG, Vazquez F, Haswell JR, Manchester HE, et al. ARID1B is a specific vulnerability in ARID1A-mutant cancers. Nature Medicine. 2014;20(3):251–254.

[133] Ogiwara H, Sasaki M, Mitachi T, Oike T, Higuchi S, Tominaga Y, et al. Targeting p300 addiction in CBP-deficient cancers causes synthetic lethality by apoptotic cell death due to abrogation of MYC expression. Cancer Discovery. 2016;6(4):430–445.

[134] Jin Q, Yu LR, Wang L, Zhang Z, Kasper LH, Lee JE, et al. Distinct roles of GCN5/PCAF-mediated H3K9ac and CBP/p300-mediated H3K18/27ac in nuclear receptor transactivation. The EMBO Journal. 2011;30(2):249–262.

[135] Tie F, Banerjee R, Stratton CA, Prasad-Sinha J, Stepanik V, Zlobin A, et al. CBP-mediated acetylation of histone H3 lysine 27 antagonizes Drosophila Polycomb silencing. Development. 2009;136(18):3131–3141.

[136] Gui Y, Guo G, Huang Y, Hu X, Tang A, Gao S, et al. Frequent mutations of chromatin remodeling genes in transitional cell carcinoma of the bladder. Nature Genetics. 2011;43(9):875–878.

[137] Morin RD, Mendez-Lago M, Mungall AJ, Goya R, Mungall KL, Corbett RD, et al. Frequent mutation of histone-modifying genes in non-Hodgkin lymphoma. Nature. 2011;476(7360):298–303.

[138] Mullighan CG, Zhang J, Kasper LH, Lerach S, Payne-Turner D, Phillips LA, et al. CREBBP mutations in relapsed acute lymphoblastic leukaemia. Nature. 2011;471(7337): 235–239.

[139] Cross NC. Histone modification defects in developmental disorders and cancer. Oncotarget. 2012;3(1):3–4.

[140] Ahuja N, Easwaran H, Baylin SB. Harnessing the potential of epigenetic therapy to target solid tumors. The Journal of Clinical Investigation. 2014;124(1):56–63.

[141] Tsai HC, Li H, Van Neste L, Cai Y, Robert C, Rassool FV, et al. Transient low doses of DNA-demethylating agents exert durable antitumor effects on hematological and epithelial tumor cells. Cancer Cell. 2012;21(3):430–446.

[142] Lai F, Jin L, Gallagher S, Mijatov B, Zhang XD, Hersey P. Histone deacetylases (HDACs) as mediators of resistance to apoptosis in melanoma and as targets for combination therapy with selective BRAF inhibitors. Advances in Pharmacology. 2012;65:27–43.

[143] Xia C, Leon-Ferre R, Laux D, Deutsch J, Smith BJ, Frees M, et al. Treatment of resistant metastatic melanoma using sequential epigenetic therapy (decitabine and panobinostat) combined with chemotherapy (temozolomide). Cancer Chemotherapy and Pharmacology. 2014;74(4):691–697.

[144] Venza M, Visalli M, Oteri R, Agliano F, Morabito S, Teti D, et al. The overriding of TRAIL resistance by the histone deacetylase inhibitor MS-275 involves c-myc up-regulation in cutaneous, uveal, and mucosal melanoma. International Immunopharmacology. 2015;28(1):313–321.

[145] Reu FJ, Bae SI, Cherkassky L, Leaman DW, Lindner D, Beaulieu N, et al. Overcoming resistance to interferon-induced apoptosis of renal carcinoma and melanoma cells by DNA demethylation. Journal of Clinical Oncology. 2006;24(23):3771–3779.

[146] Bae SI, Cheriyath V, Jacobs BS, Reu FJ, Borden EC. Reversal of methylation silencing of Apo2L/TRAIL receptor 1 (DR4) expression overcomes resistance of SK-MEL-3 and SK-MEL-28 melanoma cells to interferons (IFNs) or Apo2L/TRAIL. Oncogene. 2008;27(4): 490–498.

[147] Juergens RA, Wrangle J, Vendetti FP, Murphy SC, Zhao M, Coleman B, et al. Combination epigenetic therapy has efficacy in patients with refractory advanced non-small cell lung cancer. Cancer Discovery. 2011;1(7):598–607.

[148] Wrangle J, Wang W, Koch A, Easwaran H, Mohammad HP, Vendetti F, et al. Alterations of immune response of non-small cell lung cancer with azacytidine. Oncotarget. 2013;4(11):2067–2079.

[149] Li H, Chiappinelli KB, Guzzetta AA, Easwaran H, Yen RW, Vatapalli R, et al. Immune regulation by low doses of the DNA methyltransferase inhibitor 5-azacitidine in common human epithelial cancers. Oncotarget. 2014;5(3):587–598.

[150] Chiappinelli KB, Strissel PL, Desrichard A, Li H, Henke C, Akman B, et al. Inhibiting DNA methylation causes an interferon response in cancer via dsRNA including endogenous retroviruses. Cell. 2015;162(5):974–986.

[151] Roulois D, Loo Yau H, Singhania R, Wang Y, Danesh A, Shen SY, et al. DNA-demethylating agents target colorectal cancer cells by inducing viral mimicry by endogenous transcripts. Cell. 2015;162(5):961–973.

[152] Woods DM, Woan K, Cheng F, Wang H, Perez-Villarroel P, Lee C, et al. The antimelanoma activity of the histone deacetylase inhibitor panobinostat (LBH589) is mediated by direct tumor cytotoxicity and increased tumor immunogenicity. Melanoma Research. 2013;23(5):341–348.

[153] Woan KV, Lienlaf M, Perez-Villaroel P, Lee C, Cheng F, Knox T, et al. Targeting histone deacetylase 6 mediates a dual anti-melanoma effect: Enhanced antitumor immunity and impaired cell proliferation. Molecular Oncology. 2015;9(7):1447–1457.

[154] Chang CC, Pirozzi G, Wen SH, Chung IH, Chiu BL, Errico S, et al. Multiple structural and epigenetic defects in the human leukocyte antigen class I antigen presentation pathway in a recurrent metastatic melanoma following immunotherapy. The Journal of Biological Chemistry. 2015;290(44):26562–26575.

[155] Woods DM, Sodre AL, Villagra A, Sarnaik A, Sotomayor EM, Weber J. HDAC inhibition upregulates PD-1 ligands in melanoma and augments immunotherapy with PD-1 blockade. Cancer Immunology Research. 2015;3(12):1375–1385.

[156] Kim KH, Roberts CW. Targeting EZH2 in cancer. Nature Medicine. 2016;22(2):128–134.

[157] Ribrag V, Soria JC, Michot JM, Schmitt A, Postel-Vinay S, Bijou F, et al. Phase 1 study of tazemetostat (EPZ-6438), an inhibitor of enhancer of zeste-homolog 2 (EZH2): Preliminary safety and activity in relapsed or refractory non-hodgkin lymphoma (NHL) patients. Orlando: 57th Meeting of the American Society of Hematology: 2016 Abstract 473.

[158] DuPage M, Chopra G, Quiros J, Rosenthal WL, Morar MM, Holohan D, et al. The chromatin-modifying enzyme Ezh2 is critical for the maintenance of regulatory T cell identity after activation. Immunity. 2015;42(2):227–238.

[159] Yang XP, Jiang K, Hirahara K, Vahedi G, Afzali B, Sciume G, et al. EZH2 is crucial for both differentiation of regulatory T cells and T effector cell expansion. Scientific Reports. 2015;5:10643.

[160] Peng D, Kryczek I, Nagarsheth N, Zhao L, Wei S, Wang W, et al. Epigenetic silencing of TH1-type chemokines shapes tumour immunity and immunotherapy. Nature. 2015;527(7577):249–253.

[161] Nagarsheth N, Peng D, Kryczek I, Wu K, Li W, Zhao E, et al. PRC2 epigenetically silences Th1-type chemokines to suppress effector T-cell trafficking in colon cancer. Cancer Research. 2016;76(2):275–282.

[162] Wang CY, Filippakopoulos P. Beating the odds: BETs in disease. Trends in Biochemical Sciences. 2015;40(8):468–479.

[163] Stathis A, Zucca E, Bekradda M, Gomez-Roca C, Delord JP, de La Motte Rouge T, et al. Clinical response of carcinomas harboring the BRD4-NUT oncoprotein to the targeted bromodomain inhibitor OTX015/MK-8628. Cancer Discovery 2016;6(5):492–500.

[164] Heinemann A, Cullinane C, De Paoli-Iseppi R, Wilmott JS, Gunatilake D, Madore J, et al. Combining BET and HDAC inhibitors synergistically induces apoptosis of melanoma and suppresses AKT and YAP signaling. Oncotarget. 2015;6(25):21507–21521.

[165] Stratikopoulos EE, Dendy M, Szabolcs M, Khaykin AJ, Lefebvre C, Zhou MM, et al. Kinase and BET inhibitors together clamp inhibition of PI3K signaling and overcome resistance to therapy. Cancer Cell. 2015;27(6):837–851.

[166] Knoechel B, Roderick JE, Williamson KE, Zhu J, Lohr JG, Cotton MJ, et al. An epigenetic mechanism of resistance to targeted therapy in T cell acute lymphoblastic leukemia. Nature Genetics. 2014;46(4):364–370.

[167] Bandukwala HS, Gagnon J, Togher S, Greenbaum JA, Lamperti ED, Parr NJ, et al. Selective inhibition of CD4+ T-cell cytokine production and autoimmunity by BET protein and c-Myc inhibitors. Proceedings of the National Academy of Sciences of the United States of America. 2012;109(36):14532–14537.

[168] Mele DA, Salmeron A, Ghosh S, Huang HR, Bryant BM, Lora JM. BET bromodomain inhibition suppresses TH17-mediated pathology. The Journal of Experimental Medicine. 2013;210(11):2181–2190.

[169] Helin K, Dhanak D. Chromatin proteins and modifications as drug targets. Nature. 2013;502(7472):480–488.

[170] Sayegh J, Cao J, Zou MR, Morales A, Blair LP, Norcia M, et al. Identification of small molecule inhibitors of Jumonji AT-rich interactive domain 1B (JARID1B) histone demethylase by a sensitive high throughput screen. The Journal of Biological Chemistry. 2013;288(13):9408–9417.

[171] Ismail IH, McDonald D, Strickfaden H, Xu Z, Hendzel MJ. A small molecule inhibitor of polycomb repressive complex 1 inhibits ubiquitin signaling at DNA double-strand breaks. The Journal of Biological Chemistry. 2013;288(37):26944–26954.

[172] Picaud S, Fedorov O, Thanasopoulou A, Leonards K, Jones K, Meier J, et al. Generation of a selective small molecule inhibitor of the CBP/p300 bromodomain for leukemia therapy. Cancer Research. 2015;75(23):5106–5119.

[173] Vangamudi B, Paul TA, Shah PK, Kost-Alimova M, Nottebaum L, Shi X, et al. The SMARCA2/4 ATPase domain surpasses the bromodomain as a drug target in SWI/SNF-mutant cancers: insights from cDNA rescue and PFI-3 inhibitor studies. Cancer Research. 2015;75(18):3865–3878.

Section 3

Cell Surface Markers

Chapter 3

Glycosylation of Integrins in Melanoma Progression

Ewa Pocheć and Anna Lityńska

Additional information is available at the end of the chapter

http://dx.doi.org/10.5772/64287

Abstract

Each stage of melanoma development from transformed melanocytes to metastatic lesions requires the involvement of cell adhesion receptors, among which integrins are of particular importance. Strong N-glycosylation of αβ integrin heterodimers influences their processing, activation, and functions related to the modulation of cell adhesion to extracellular matrix proteins (ECM) and the basement membrane. A lack of N-glycans on integrin chains significantly reduces their interactions with the ECM. Melanoma progression is accompanied by changes in the composition of N-glycans on integrin subunits. The glycosylation profile of integrins depends on the stage of melanoma development and on the location of the metastasis. Enhanced expression of β1,6-branched complex-type oligosaccharides and altered sialylation are well-characterized changes in the N-glycosylation of integrins observed in melanoma progression. This chapter summarizes the current state of knowledge about α3β1, α5β1, and αvβ3 integrin glycosylation in melanoma and the functional consequences of changed glycosylation for the development of this cancer.

Keywords: integrin, N-glycosylation, melanoma, β1,6 branching, migration, extracellular matrix proteins

1. Introduction

Melanoma progression and the acquisition of invasive and metastatic competence by melanoma cells are accompanied not only by changes in integrin expression but also by alterations of the sugar component of these heavily N-glycosylated adhesive proteins [1]. This post-translational modification is critical to integrin functions, mainly its interactions with extracellular matrix proteins (ECM) and the basement membrane [2]. Changes in the expression and glycosylation of integrins contribute to each stage of melanoma progression.

Human cutaneous melanoma develops in a series of definable stages, from the common acquired nevus and dysplastic nevus through the radial growth phase (RGP) and vertical growth phase (VGP) of primary melanoma and finally metastatic melanoma. During these multistep transformations, melanoma cells acquire the ability to invade the dermis and then disseminate throughout the body via blood and lymphatic vessels [3–8]. Adjustment of integrin glycosylation is an important feature of the melanoma cell's adaptation to the constantly changing conditions of its microenvironment. This chapter reviews the current state of knowledge about integrin glycosylation in the course of melanoma progression.

2. Overall characteristics of integrins

The term "integrins" introduced by Hynes reflects the capacity of these cell surface receptors to integrate ECM proteins with the cytoskeleton and with intracellular signaling pathways by physical connection [9]. The role of integrin-mediated adhesion to the ECM in cell survival is now accepted. Integrins are heterodimeric cell surface adhesion molecules consisting of α and β subunits. By combining 18 α with 8 β subunits, at least 24 integrin dimers can be formed, each with its own characteristic specificity for ligands [10] (**Figure 1**).

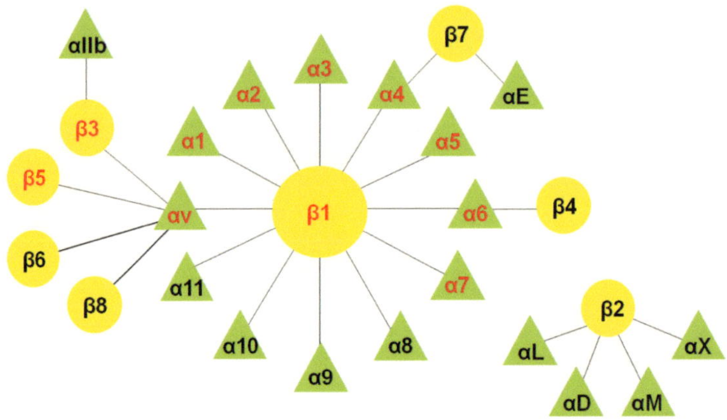

Figure 1. Integrin classification based on β subunits possessed in common. Integrin heterodimers whose expression was observed to increase during melanoma progression are marked in red.

2.1. The structure of α and β subunit ectodomains

Each integrin subunit consists of a large extracellular domain and short transmembrane and cytoplasmic domains. The extracellular domains (ectodomains) of the α and β subunits are constructed of several subdomains joined together by flexible linkers [11, 12]. The crystal structure of the $\alpha v\beta 3$ [13] and $\alpha IIb\beta 3$ [14] ectodomains has been characterized in detail.

The ectodomain of the α-subunit contains four or five elements: a seven-bladed β-propeller, a thigh, and two calfs. There are also nine integrins with an α-subunit containing an additional α-I domain inserted between blades 2 and 3 of the β-propeller. A structure similar to an α-I domain is also present in the β subunit of integrins. The β-propeller contains Ca^{2+}-binding sites needed for ligand binding. The thigh and calf of the α-subunit have 140–170 residues folded into an immunoglobulin-like domain.

The ectodomain of the β-subunit consists of seven subdomains: a PSI (plexin-semaphorin-integrin), an Ig-like hybrid, a β-I-like domain, and four EGF-like modules (epidermal growth factor-like modules), followed by the β-tail part. The β-I-like domain is inserted into the hybrid modules and shows homology to the α-I domain. The PSI domain is split into two parts. The α-I domain is the primary region of ligand binding in integrins that have this structure, whereas the other integrins form the binding site through the cooperation of both subunit ectodomains (β-propeller/β-I-like interface) [15]. It has been suggested that the I-domain can exist as an "open" (high-affinity) or "closed" (low-affinity) conformation. The presence of a "metal-ion-dependent-adhesion-site" (MIDAS) motif indicates the role of divalent metal ions in achievement of the high-affinity state by integrins.

The transmembrane segments of each subunit are followed by a short cytoplasmic tail. Although they have no enzymatic activity, cytoplasmic tails play an important role in integrin activity and signal transfer.

2.2. Bidirectional signaling of integrins

Integrins are involved in bidirectional signaling—inside-out and outside-in—through their function as a linker between the ECM and the cytoskeleton [16, 17]. Control of the integrin conformation state is required for their signaling. There is little agreement among the findings from nuclear magnetic resonance (NMR) studies of cytoplasmic tails [12], but other data support the view that transmembrane and cytoplasmic domains play a key role in this signaling. In the inactive state, these domains are closely associated; separation of the chain results in activation of adhesion [11, 16].

Inside-out activation is mediated by talin binding to the β-tail, which interrupts the α/β interaction [18]. In fact, a large number of proteins have been shown to interact with cytoplasmic domains of integrins, among them cytoskeleton proteins (talin, filamin, and kindlins), adaptor proteins, and kinases [11, 19]. Talin and kindlins bound to β-integrin cooperate to regulate integrin affinity [19]. Upon binding of the ligand to the integrins' extracellular domain, signal transduction to the cytoplasm is transmitted in the classical direction: outside-in. Generation of intracellular signals leads to the formation of a focal adhesion complex which involves over 150 intracellular proteins and serves as a center of intracellular signaling [20]. Among these proteins are scaffolding molecules and also kinases such as focal adhesion kinase (FAK) and Src family kinase (SFK). So the function of integrin is related to its ligand affinity, which can be induced either by conformational changes or by clustering on the cell surface [11].

2.3. Classification of integrins and their ligands

The first classification of integrins was based on the presence of a common β subunit having distinct α subfamilies. Recent work has shown that one α subunit may associate with different β subunits, in particular a αv subunit. However, the largest number of integrins are still assigned to the β1 (VLA, very late-activated antigens) subfamily. In this group, are integrins recognizing fibronectin (FN) (α5β1, α4β1), collagen (α1β1, α2β1, α10β1, α11β1) or laminin (LN) (α2β1, α3β1, α6β1, α7β1) [21, 22] (**Figure 1**). The α4β1 integrin present on human lymphocytes has been shown to bind vascular cell adhesion molecule 1 (VCAM-1), the cell surface protein of activated endothelia. The β2 subfamily of integrins is limited to white blood cells. Recognition of cell surface receptors of the Ig superfamily by β2 integrins is crucial to leukocyte–endothelium interaction [22, 23]. The β3 subfamily consists of two members: platelet receptor (αIIbβ3) and vitronectin - receptor (αvβ3). Integrin αIIbβ3 is specific for platelets; it recognizes fibrinogen specifically but upon platelet activation can also bind fibronectin (FN), von Willebrand's factor and thrombospondin. Integrin αvβ3 binds multiple ligands including vitronectin (VN), fibrinogen, thrombospondin, and von Willebrand's factor [23]. αv subunit can associate with more than one β subunit, such as β1, β5, β6, and β8 [22].

Integrins bind to a specific motif in their ligands. The RGD (Arg-Gly-Asp) sequence found within matrix proteins including FN, VN, thrombospondin, and laminin (LN) is usually recognized by integrins [12, 23], but there are integrins that recognize their ligands through motifs other than RGD. Integrins, α3β1, α6β1, and α7β1, being highly specific LN receptors, bind to different regions of this ligand [12]. Fibrinogen contains the binding sequence Lys-Gln-Ala-Gly-Asp-Val, while Asp-Gly-Glu-Ala was found to be the dominant binding motif in type I collagen [24].

3. Integrin expression in melanoma

Changes in integrin expression have been studied extensively in melanoma carcinogenesis [8, 25]. The integrin profile of melanoma cells differs significantly from that of normal melanocytes [26, 27] and is closely related to the stage of melanoma progression [24, 28]. Flow cytometry showed significant differences in the expression of α2, α3, β1, and especially α5 integrin subunits between WM35 primary and two metastatic human cell lines (WM9 and A375), indicating that acceleration of melanoma invasion is accompanied by increased integrin subunit synthesis [29]. Significant up-regulation of α5 integrin expression was also shown in highly metastatic B16-F10 murine melanoma cells as compared to weakly metastatic B16-F1 cells [30]. A low level of α3β1 integrin was found in benign lesions of primary melanoma, whereas in malignant cutaneous melanoma, the expression of the heterodimer progressively increased and was connected with the degree of invasion into the dermis [31].

It is well documented in *in vitro* models that melanoma development and acquisition of the metastatic phenotype are also correlated with the expression of αvβ3 integrin [26, 32, 33]. An early study by Albelda et al. [34] showed that the β3 subunit is restricted to the VGP and metastatic melanomas; in the RGP and in nevus cells, this integrin chain was not found. A study of pairs of differing melanoma cells taken from the same patient (primary WM115 and metastatic WM266-4 cell lines) supported previous observations that in primary melanoma the cells survive without αv integrins, while in disease progression, their growth and functions depend on this receptor's expression [35]. Our group detected αvβ3 integrin in both primary RGP-derived (WM35) and metastatic melanoma cells (WM9, WM239 and A397 cell lines) [36, 37]. On the other hand, immunohistochemical staining of αvβ3 in human tumor tissue samples did not confirm a positive correlation of integrin expression with the melanoma metastatic phenotype; melanoma *in situ* with a pre-invasive phenotype showed the highest level of αvβ3 expression [38].

Most studies have demonstrated up-regulation of integrin expression in melanoma carcinogenesis; only a few integrin receptors have been found to reduce their expression during disease progression. Ziober et al. [39] found that acquisition of a highly metastatic phenotype by melanoma cells was accompanied by loss of α7β1 expression.

Enhancement of the expression of most integrins promotes conversion of melanoma from the RGP to the VGP and then acquisition of metastatic competence. The switch in expression from LN-binding to FN-binding integrins was shown to contribute to the movement of melanoma cells from the epidermis to the dermis through degraded basement membrane. Apart from induction of αvβ3 expression, the involvement of α3β1 [31], α5β1, and αvβ5 integrins in this process has been found [40].

4. Functions of integrins: role of glycosylation

Integrins participate in a wide range of biological processes, including growth, proliferation, differentiation, survival/apoptosis, and cell-cycle regulation [41–44]. Apart from the adhesion function, they mediate cell signaling events [45–47].

Tumor progression requires comprehensive alteration of normal cell-cell and cell-ECM interactions [34, 48]. Integrins are the main adhesion proteins responsible for these changes, mainly due to their altered expression. They contribute to regulation of such processes as angiogenesis, tumor growth and metastasis, as well as cell proliferation, survival and motility [49–53]. Abundant glycosylation of the extracellular domains of integrins also significantly affects the function of these receptors [2, 54, 55].

Glycosylation is one of the most frequent post-translational modifications of transmembrane and secreted proteins. Both integrin chains are subject to this modification [56]. Integrin α subunits are more profusely N-glycosylated than their β partners. Subunits α3, α5, and αv in the polypeptide sequences contain 13, 14, and 13 potential N-glycosylation sites, respectively, whereas the β1 and β3 chains include 12 and 6 N-glycan-linked sequences, respectively [57]. Intensive glycosylation of integrin chains during post-translational processing results in high content of the sugar component of the whole glycoprotein molecule. Peptide N-glycosidase F (PNGase F) digestion showed that ca. 24 and 25% of the glycoprotein's molecular weight (MW) responds to N-glycans in α3 subunits from WM35 primary and A375 metastatic melanoma cells, respectively. N-oligosaccharides on β1 subunits account for ca. 24 and 33% of total MW in primary and metastatic cells, respectively. In both subunits, the pool of sialic acids increases in metastatic cells in compared with primary melanoma [58] (**Figure 2**). N-oligosaccharides on the αv integrin subunit from WM793 primary melanoma cells respond to nearly 30% of glycoprotein MW, and from WM1205Lu metastatic cells 28%. Subunit β3 contains 16% of the N-glycans in WM793 cells and 12% of the N-glycans in WM1205Lu cells [59].

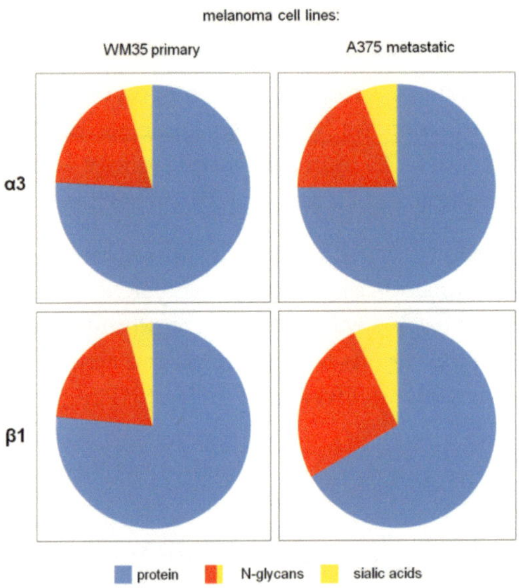

Figure 2. Percentage content of the N-glycan pool and sialic acid in subunits of α3β1 integrin, based on Pocheć et al. [58].

Integrin chains bear all types of N-glycan structures, starting from the evolutionarily oldest structures high-mannose-type, through hybrid glycans, and ending in the most complicated complex-type oligosaccharides [1, 54]. The occurrence of these glycostructures on β1 integrins in B16-F10 melanoma cells depends on the stage of integrin maturation. High-mannose glycans recognized by GNA lectin (*Galanthus nivalis* agglutinin) were abundant on the immature form of β1 integrins with lower molecular weight. The mature, larger β1 chain carried mostly sialylated complex-type structures, identified using DSA (*Datura stramonium* agglutinin) and MAA (*Maackia ammurensis* agglutinin) lectins. Only the completely processed form of β1 integrin was detected at the cell surface of murine melanoma [60].

Glycosylation is crucial to the processing, activation, and functioning of integrins [56, 61]. The function of integrin glycans has been determined mostly using N-glycan synthesis inhibitors, such as castanospermine and N-methyldeoxynojirimycin, which block glucosidases I and II responsible for trimming glucose from the precursor form of N-linked oligosaccharides; 1-deoxymannojirimycin and swainsonine (SW), inhibitors of mannosidase I and II, respectively, and tunicamycin, which abolishes N-glycosylation by inhibiting the action of N-acetylglucosamine-1-phosphotransferase. Other useful tools for assessing N-glycan functioning are recombinant glycosidases, such as PNGase F, which removes glycans N-linked to the protein backbone, and endo-N-acetylglucosaminidase F (Endo F), which cleaves high-mannose and complex-type N-glycans [62].

Glycosylation of αvβ3 integrin is necessary to assembly of the heterodimer, proteolytic cleavage of the α chain, and cell surface expression of this VN receptor in human melanoma cells. Application of castanospermine and N-methyldeoxynojirimycin decreased αvβ3 surface expression as the result of reduced chain assembly and α polypeptide cleavage. On the other hand, 1-deoxymannojirimycin and SW, inhibitors acting on the later stages of glycan synthesis, did not influence αvβ3 transport to the cell membrane [63]. The importance of N-glycosylation in associating the two subunits was also clearly demonstrated by treating α5βl integrin with Endo F and PNGase F. Enzymatic digestion of purified α5βl integrin resulted in separate precipitation of the α and β polypeptide chains; undigested integrin subunits underwent co-precipitation [64]. Further research using sequential side-directed mutagenesis showed that N-glycosylation of the I-like domain of the βl subunit is essential for the formation of the α5βl heterodimer and for integrin functioning [65].

Cell surface carbohydrates present on adhesion proteins are involved in adhesive and migratory events crucial to each step of the metastatic process. In early studies by Chammas et al., it was found that glycosylation of the β1 subunit complexed with α6 integrin is essential for interaction with LN. Binding of B16-F10 melanoma cells to LN via α6βl integrin was nearly abolished in tunicamycin-treated cells and after treating LN with Endo F/PNGase F [66]. Similarly, digestion of α5βl integrin with a mixture of Endo F and PNGase F led to the loss of FN binding [64]. Lectin analysis showed that both subunits of α6βl integrin bear mainly sialylated complex-type N-glycan structures. Exoglycosidase treatment identified galactose residues on the α subunit as the LN-binding determinants involved in cell adhesion to this ECM ligand. The integrin β chain, abundant in complex-type structures, whose synthesis was inhibited by SW (which blocks the formation of complex-type glycans, among them β1,6-branched glycans), was associated with cell spread but not cell adhesion [67]. Also, human metastatic malignant melanoma cell lines LOX and FEMX treated with tunicamycin showed significantly weaker adhesion to LN and to a lesser extent to type IV collagen. Inhibition of N-glycan synthesis by tunicamycin resulted in reduction of LOX and FEMX invasion through Matrigel-coated chambers, as well as diminution of human melanoma aggregation [68].

5. Alterations of integrin glycosylation in melanoma carcinogenesis

The vast majority of studies on integrin glycosylation in melanoma have used mouse melanoma cell line B16-F10 and phenotypic variants of it that show different degrees of invasive potential, mainly the weakly invasive cell lines B16-F1 or B16-Flr, and B16-BL6 cells selected for their higher ability to metastasize to the lungs [60, 67, 69–73], as well as human melanoma cell lines derived from each stage of melanoma progression, most of which were established by Herlyn's group [3].

It has been demonstrated that the glycosylation profile of integrins depends on the stage of melanoma development [37, 58, 59, 74] and the location of the metastasis [75, 76] and that glycosylation is essential to the interaction between integrin and ECM proteins during adhesion and migration processes [58, 75, 76]. These studies have produced ample evidence for the presence of glycoforms associated with melanoma carcinogenesis on α3β1, α5β1, and αvβ3 integrins. The changes in the β1,6 branching of complex-type N-glycans, and their sialylation, have been observed on these integrins during human melanoma progression.

5.1. Branched complex-type N-glycans

One of the well-characterized changes in N-glycosylation is enhanced expression of β1,6-N-acetylglucosaminyltransferase V (GnT-V) and its products, N-acetylglucosamine (GlcNAc) β1,6-branched N-linked oligosaccharides, observed in the tumorigenesis of many cancers [77–81], including melanoma [74]. β1,6-branched N-glycans are important in invasion of the basement membrane [82] and acquisition of metastatic competence [83]. β1,6 branching of glycans on integrin chains has been described in studies of mouse and human melanoma.

The presence of β1,6-branched complex-type oligosaccharides on the integrin receptors that bind LN and FN was first shown by Chammas et al. in mouse melanoma cell line B16-F10 [70] and then confirmed on the β1 subunit sharing integrins in this parent cell line and its highly invasive B16-BL6 variant [73, 84, 85]. Significantly enhanced β1,6 branching found on highly invasive B16-BL6 cells resulted in their more efficient invasion and migration, as well as impaired adhesion to different ECM proteins (LN, FN, VN, type I and type IV collagen, hyaluronic acid, and Matrigel). Inhibition of β1,6 branching on two levels—expression of GnT-V by cell transfection (using antisense cDNA), and oligosaccharide synthesis (using SW)—decreased metastasis and invasion of B16-BL6 cells by half, and reduced the formation of metastatic colonies in lungs [73]. Later it was found that α3β1 and α5β1 integrins on mouse B16-BL6 cells carry β1,6-branched oligosaccharides and that β1,6-glycosylation of integrins has an effect on the spread of melanoma cells on FN and Matrigel. Interestingly, β1,6-branched glycans on α3β1 weakened the association of integrin with CD151 tetraspanin [85]. Earlier the crucial role of glycosylation in the interaction of α3β1 with CD151 had been described in work using MDA-MB-231 human breast cancer cells [86]. For B16-BL6 mouse melanoma cells, it was shown (by co-precipitating α3β1 and CD151 from SW-treated cells) that β1,6-branched N-glycans regulate the association of CD151 with this integrin [85].

In human melanoma cells, we demonstrated β1,6 branching of cancer-associated integrin subunits such as α2, α3, α4, α5, αv, β1, and β3 [37]; integrin heterodimers of special importance in melanoma carcinogenesis are α3β1 [58, 75], α5β1 [74], and αvβ3 [59, 75, 87].

A number of studies have confirmed the involvement of α3β1 integrin in melanoma development through its participation in cell adhesion, migration, and invasion [88–90]. The ability of α3β1 to promote melanoma metastasis results from its enhanced synthesis [91, 92] and also from altered glycosylation of it, particularly enhanced β1,6 branching [58, 74, 75].

Glycosylation of α3β1 integrin was first recognized as a factor promoting tumorigenesis in human colon carcinoma cells. Sialylated β1,6-branched Asn-linked oligosaccharides with short poly-N-acetyllactosamine units were found on both integrin subunits. Due to their role in cancer development, they were suggested to be oncodevelopmental carbohydrate epitopes [93].

Different techniques have been employed to analyze α3β1 integrin glycosylation in detail in melanoma cells derived from primary and metastatic tumors. The use of matrix-assisted laser desorption/ionization mass spectrometry (MALDI-MS) showed the presence of tetra-antennary complex-type glycans on the β1 subunit in highly metastatic A375 melanoma cells but not in WM35 cells from the primary site. The reaction of affinity-chromatography-purified α3β1 integrin with *Phaseolus vulgaris* agglutinin (PHA-L) revealed that complex-type glycans are β1,6-branched in the α3 subunit from metastatic but not from primary cells [58]. The presence of GlcNAc β1,6-branched glycans on α3β1 in A375 metastatic cells was confirmed by tandem mass spectrometry (MS/MS) of PHA-L-positive glycoproteins eluted in lectin-affinity chromatography [36]. The absence of this type of branching on the α3 subunit in WM35 primary melanoma was thoroughly documented by MS/MS identification of PHA-L bound proteins and two-sided control of integrin glycosylation: immunoblotting in PHA-L-eluted material and PHA-L blotting in immunoprecipitation [37]. In two other metastatic melanoma cell lines (WM9 and WM239), β1,6 branching of α3β1 integrin was shown using MS/MS identification of PHA-L-bound glycoproteins [37] and confirmed using MALDI-MS and PHA-L precipitation [75]. The amount of glycans with β1,6-linked antenna increased in WM1205Lu metastatic melanoma as compared to WM793 primary cells [74]. Using normal-phase high-performance liquid chromatography (NP-HPLC), however, Link-Lenczowski et al. [94] did not observe differences in α3β1 glycosylation profiles between WM115 primary and WM266-4 metastatic human melanoma cell lines originating from the same patient.

The role of α5 integrin in promoting melanoma metastasis has been shown in uveal [95] and cutaneous melanoma [29, 96]. An increase of the metastatic potential of melanoma is accompanied by enhancement of α5 integrin expression [30, 97]. In highly metastatic B16-F10 melanoma cells, the level of α5 integrin was conspicuously elevated as compared to weakly metastatic B16-F1 cells. Pulmonary metastasis in mice as well as the adhesion and spread of B16-F10 cells to FN *in vitro* was significantly reduced after blocking of α5 integrin by a specific antibody. The loss of α5-mediated melanoma cell-FN anchoring promoted apoptosis of B16-F10 cells [30].

Integrin α5β1 is also a carrier of β1,6-branched glycans in metastatic cells, but on the α5 subunit from primary melanoma, this type of branching was not detected. In each of three analyzed metastatic cell lines (WM9, WM239 and A375), the α5 subunit oligosaccharides were β1,6-branched [37], but not the α5 chain in WM35 melanoma cells [36], as determined using MS/MS analysis of PHA-L-positive glycoproteins. A comparison of α5 integrin chains from early VGP and metastatic lesion cells showed an uptrend of β1,6 branching during acquisition of metastatic competence [74]. These findings suggest that GlcNAc β1,6-branched structures appear earlier in melanoma development on the β1 subunit than on the α3 and α5 chains and that in melanoma cancerogenesis their content is more stable on the β1 subunit than on the α3 and α5 chains [36, 37, 74].

Glycosylation of integrin αvβ3 is still rather poorly understood [54], although it is well known that this integrin is associated with the metastatic potential of melanoma [33, 35, 98]. Our studies using two genetically related melanoma cell lines showed the presence of β1,6-branched complex-type structures on primary and metastatic cells, but we did not observe differences in the β1,6 branching of αvβ3 glycans during the transition from primary VGP melanoma to its metastatic variant. PHA-L precipitation and SW treatment gave similar levels of β1,6 branching in both αvβ3 subunits in cell lines WM793 and WM1205Lu [59]. This type of glycan was also present on the αv subunit from RGP-derived WM35 melanoma cells, but β1,6 branching was not found on the β3 chain from these cells [36]. Integrin αvβ3 from three metastatic cell lines (WM9, WM239 and A375) of varying origin showed expression of these structures [37, 75].

The phenomenon of competition for a substrate between N-acetylglucosaminyltransferase III (GnT-III) and GnT-V is well documented in N-glycan biology. GnT-III activity during N-glycan processing can suppress the biological functions of GnT-V; it results in reduction of N-glycan β1,6 branching. With respect to integrins, this was first shown on α3β1 in human gastric cancer cell line MKN45 [99]. In B16 melanoma cells, ectopic expression of GnT-III was shown to retard cell metastasis through inhibition of GnT-V activity: the absence of GnT-V products was associated with attenuation of malignant cell motility [83]. Our group showed a significant decrease of bisecting GlcNAc content on αvβ3 integrin subunits during the transition from the VGP to the metastatic stage, but it was not associated with any change in the amount of β1,6-branched glycans on this integrin [59], although previously in this pair of related cell lines (WM115 vs. WM1205Lu), we observed significant upregulation of GnT-V expression [74].

Integrin-mediated cell migration requires adhesion of cells to ECM substrates and is essential for dissemination of the tumor to distant organs during metastasis [100], so the role of integrin glycosylation is frequently assessed in different adhesion and migration tests. Functional studies have clearly shown that β1,6 branching on cell surface adhesion receptors, mainly integrins, promotes melanoma cell migration [101], and invasion [90].

The contribution of α3β1 integrin's N-glycans to its binding with its ECM ligands was demonstrated using affinity-chromatography-purified integrin from WM35 primary and A375 metastatic melanoma cells. In direct ligand-binding assays, de-N-glycosylated α3β1 integrin showed enhanced binding of both melanoma cell lines to LN, type IV collagen and FN, except for the binding of α3β1 from WM35 to FN [58]. Enzymatic removal of N-glycans from this integrin in two metastatic melanoma cell lines from metastases of different origin (WM9 and WM239) also resulted in enhanced binding of α3β1 to LN5 [75].

Of the ECM proteins, fibronectin is the major α5β1 ligand [102] and therefore is the one most frequently chosen for assays evaluating the involvement of α5β1 integrin in adhesion and migration processes. β1,6 branching of FN receptors was shown to contribute to migration of metastatic melanoma on FN, but not to primary cell migration [74].

N-glycan-dependent binding of integrins to the ECM triggers intracellular pathways via phosphorylation of cytoplasmic kinases. FAK is one of the first proteins recruited to integrins aggregated within the cell membrane. Activation of signal pathways leads to the expression of different genes that control cell growth, differentiation, tumor invasion and metastasis [103, 104]. Changes in integrin glycosylation affect intracellular signals triggered by melanoma cell binding to the ECM. Dual immunostaining of melanoma cells growing on VN showed co-localization of αvβ3 integrin and FAK, a downstream target of integrins, in focal adhesion sites of melanoma cells. Overexpression of GnT-V in human WM266-4 metastatic melanoma cells up-regulated αvβ3-integrin-mediated FAK phosphorylation and cell migration on VN, while inhibition of β1,6 branching by SW-treatment reduced FAK signaling activation in both A375 and WM266-4 metastatic cells [87].

An interesting aspect of integrin glycans' involvement in melanoma metastasis is their participation in ECM degradation through regulation of the activity of matrix proteases, such as urokinase-type plasminogen activator (uPA) and metalloproteinases (MMPs). Integrins interact with urokinase-type plasminogen activator receptors (uPARs) in the cell membrane [105]. A urokinase-type plasminogen activator (uPA), acting via its receptor (uPAR), catalyzes the activation of plasmin from plasminogen, and the plasmin initiates a proteolytic cascade leading to degradation of the ECM [106, 107]. Our work demonstrated that β1,6-branched oligosaccharides on αvβ3 and α3β1 integrins are essential for the association of the uPAR with integrins in human melanoma cell lines WM9 and WM239, seen in the failure of co-precipitation of the two integrins with the uPAR in SW-treated cells. Adhesion of the two melanoma cells to VN was dependant on β1,6 branching of αvβ3 and α3β1 integrins in a cell-line-specific manner [76].

N-glycans with β1,6-branched antennae on melanoma integrins also modify the activity of metalloproteinases (MMPs). PHA-L precipitation revealed that β1 integrins from B16-BL6 cells are more β1,6-branched than the parent cells with lower invasion ability. β1,6-glycosylation of β1 integrin receptors affected the activation of membrane-tethered forms of metalloproteinases (MT1-MMPs). The association of β1,6-glycosylation-suppressed β1 integrin with MT1-MMPs was more severely affected in B16-BL6 cells than in the parent cells, suggesting that integrin β1,6 branching contributes to melanoma invasion also through activation of MMPs [84].

5.2. Sialylation

Sialic acid-linked α2,3 or α2,6, mostly in terminal positions of the oligosaccharide, gives these molecules a negative charge [108, 109] that significantly influences cell interaction mediated by sialylated adhesion proteins, among them integrins [110]. Hypersialylation of cell surface receptors is important in tumor invasion and metastasis [111]. MAA is the lectin commonly used to analyze a pool of α2,3-linked sialic acid, while a lectin from *Sambucus nigra* (SNA) is specific for α2,6-linked sialic acid [112]. The presence of sialic acids on α3β1, α5β1, and αvβ3 integrins in melanoma cells was confirmed in each stage of melanoma progression [58, 59, 75].

One of the first studies on integrin sialylation in melanoma employed mouse melanoma cell lines differing in their metastatic ability. Analysis of melanoma cell sialylation using HPLC and digestion by *Vibrio cholerae* sialidase did not show changes in the total content of cell surface sialic acids on mouse B16 metastatic melanoma cell variants differing in their invasive potential [69]. Research on specific adhesion proteins provided more detailed information. Integrin β1 from both B16-F1 mouse metastatic melanoma and its weakly metastatic wheat germ agglutinin-resistant mutant Wa4-b1 was found to contain high-mannose and bi-, tri-, and tetra-antennary complex-type N-oligosaccharides. Sialylation of the β1 subunit was significantly decreased in mutant melanoma cells with low metastatic ability. Alteration of β1 integrin glycosylation resulted in reduction of the mutant's metastatic potential and adhesion to FN and LN, as compared to the parent cells [71]. Higher β1,6 branching of complex-type glycans on more invasive B16-BL6 melanoma cells versus the parent B16-F10 line was correlated with an increase of α2,3-linked and α2,6-linked sialic acid content as determined using MAA and SNA staining in flow cytometry. Hypersialylation of B16-BL6 cells resulted in their higher motility and stronger adhesion to selected ECM proteins [73]. Further results for this pair of murine melanoma cell lines were obtained by lectin blotting: α2,6-linked sialic acid especially increased on B16-BL6 glycans as a result of enhanced β1,6 branching. α2,6-desialylation and down-regulation of the sialyltransferase ST6Gal-I, which transfers sialic acids to oligosaccharides and catalyzes the formation of α2,6 linkage, negatively affected adhesion and invasion of B16-BL6 cells [113]. In turn, a study by Chang and colleagues showed that α2,3-linked sialic acid is important in the metastasis of B16-F10 cells. Soyasaponin I (Ssa I), which specifically inhibits the expression of α2,3-linked sialic acids, reduced the migratory ability of melanoma, up-regulated cell adhesion to ECM proteins, and impaired pulmonary metastasis [114].

Our studies using different human melanoma cell line models indicated reduction of α2,3 sialylation on the α3 integrin subunit, and of α2,6 sialylation on αvβ3 integrin, in melanoma progression [74, 59]. Lectin-probed Western blotting showed that the β1 subunit from both cell lines and the α3 subunit from primary melanoma cell line WM35 had both types of sialic acid linkage, while the α3 subunit from metastatic cell line A375 lost its α2,3 glycosidic linkage [58]. Using genetically matched cell lines WM793 and WM1205Lu from the last two stages of melanoma progression, we observed a shift in the sialylation of αvβ3 integrin during the transition from VGP to metastatic tumor. Lectin MAA and SNA precipitation as well as digestion by two neuraminidases with narrower (α2,3) and wider (α2-3,6,8) specificity showed that α2,6-linked sialic acid was reduced, whereas α2,3-linked sialic acid increased on both integrin subunits from metastatic lesion cells. In a wound-healing assay, migration of melanoma cells on VN in the presence of both lectins was affected only in the metastatic cell line [59]. Lectin flow cytometry of another pair of related melanoma cell lines (WM115 derived from RGP/VGP vs. WM266-4 from lymph node metastasis) indicated a more than fourfold increase of cell surface α2,3 sialylation during the acquisition of metastatic competence. Despite these differences in surface α2,3 sialylation, the reduction of migration by MAA-treated primary and melanoma cells was comparable, suggesting the involvement of receptor(s) other than αvβ3 integrin and its/their sialylation in metastatic cell migration (data not published).

Digestion of α3β1 glycans with a broad-specificity neuraminidase from *Arthrobacter ureafaciens* led to stronger binding of the integrin to various ECM components (LN, FN, and type IV collagen) in both primary and metastatic melanoma cells. Interestingly, removal of the sialic acids by neuraminidase enhanced integrin binding significantly more than complete de-N-glycosylation did, suggesting an important role of desialylated N-oligosaccharides in integrin-ECM interactions [58]. For efficient cell-ECM adhesion, protein-protein interactions apparently are not enough, and glycosylation is needed to regulate this binding.

Attachment of α2,8 to underlying glycans by sialic acid is rather rarely detected on integrins. A study using human melanoma cell line G361 is one of the few that have demonstrated the presence of α2,8-bound sialic acid on α5β1 integrin—and the role of this type of sialylation in FN binding. Desialylation using an enzyme from *Arthrobacter ureafaciens* specific for α2-3,6,8-linked sialic acids resulted in reduction of α5β1-mediated adhesion to FN, an effect not observed for neuraminidase, which cleaves only α2-3,6 linkages [115].

Undoubtedly, the sialylation state of integrins contributes to the metastatic potential of mouse and human melanoma, but there are blank spots in our understanding of the role of α2,3-linked and α2,6-linked sialic acid in melanoma progression. Further studies should establish precisely how sialylation becomes altered, and its contribution to the disease phenotype.

6. Conclusions

The search for glyco-biomarkers on integrins in melanoma progression motivates a host of studies performed by different research groups. Identification of universally present alterations of glycans on adhesion molecules, among them integrins—and elucidation of the molecular mechanisms of these changes—will boost our understanding of how melanoma cells acquire the ability to escape the primary tumor and spread through the body. Enhanced β1,6 branching and altered sialylation are the main glyco-features of integrin glycosylation in melanoma progression. The functional consequences of surface glycosylation rearrangements in melanoma progression must be known if we are to find effective ways to stop the process of carcinogenesis. The vast majority of studies on integrin glycosylation in melanoma cells have used cells cultured *in vitro*. A hugely important task for future research is to verify the results obtained from *in vitro* studies of tumor tissue from patients with melanoma, so that those findings can be applied for prevention and treatment of melanoma.

Author details

Ewa Pocheć* and Anna Lityńska

*Address all correspondence to: ewa.pochec@uj.edu.pl

Department of Glycoconjugate Biochemistry, Institute of Zoology, Jagiellonian University, Krakow, Poland

References

[1] Link-Lenczowski P, Lityńska A. Glycans in melanoma screening. Part 2. Towards the understanding of integrin N-glycosylation in melanoma. Biochem Soc Trans. 2011;39(1):374–377. doi:10.1042/BST0390374

[2] Gu J, Taniguchi N. Potential of N-glycan in cell adhesion and migration as either a positive or negative regulator. Cell Adh Migr. 2008;2(4):243–245. doi:10.4161/cam. 2.4.67.48

[3] Herlyn M. Human melanoma: development and progression. Cancer Metastasis Rev. 1990;9(2):101–112. doi:10.1007/BF00046337

[4] Seftor RE, Seftor EA, Hendrix MJ. Molecular role(s) for integrins in human melanoma invasion. Cancer Metastasis Rev. 1999;18(3):359–375. doi:10.1023/A:1006317125454

[5] McGary EC, Lev DC, Bar-Eli M. Cellular adhesion pathways and metastatic potential of human melanoma. Cancer Biol Ther. 2002;1(5):459–465. doi:104161/cbt.1.5.158

[6] Satyamoorthy K, Herlyn M. Cellular and molecular biology of human melanoma. Cancer Biol Ther. 2002;1(1):14–17. doi:10.4161/cbt.1.1.32

[7] Chudnovsky Y, Khavari PA, Adams AE. Melanoma genetics and the development of rational therapeutics. J Clin Invest. 2005;115(4):813–824. doi:10.1172/JCI24808

[8] Monteiro AC, Toricelli M, Jasiulionis MG. Signaling pathways altered during the metastatic progression of melanoma. In: Murph M. editor. Current clinical management and future therapeutics. InTech; 2015. p. 49–78. doi:10.5772/59747

[9] Hynes RO. Integrins: a family of cell surface receptors. Cell. 1987;48:549–554. doi: 10.1016/0092-8674(87)90233-9

[10] Desgrosellier JS, Cheresh DA. Integrins in cancer: biological implications and therapeutic opportunities. Nat Rev Cancer. 2010;10(1):9–22. doi:10.1038/nrc2748

[11] Gahmberg CG, Fagerholm SC, Nurmi SM, Chavakis T, Marcheas S, Gronhold M. Regulation of integrin activity and signaling. Biochim. Biophys. Acta. 2009;1790(6):431–444. doi:10.1016/j.bbagen.2009.03.007

[12] Cambell ID, Humphries MJ. Integrin structure, activation, and interactions. Cold Spring Harb Perspect Biol. 2011;3(3). pii:a004994. doi:10.1101/cshperspect.a004994

[13] Xiong JP, Stehle T, Zhang R, Joachimiak A, Frech M, Goodman SL, Arnaout MA. Crystal structure of the extracellular segment of integrin $\alpha v\beta 3$ in complex with an Arg-Gly-Asp ligand. Science. 2002;296:151–155. doi:10.1126/science.1069040

[14] Zhu J, Luo BH, Xiao T, Zhang C, Nishida N, Springer TA. Structure of a complete integrin ectodomain in a physiologic resting state and activation and deactivation by applied forces. Mol Cell. 2008;32:849–861. doi:10.1016/j.molcel.2008.11.018

[15] Xiong JP, Stehle T, Diefenbach B, Zhang R, Dunker R, Scott DL, Joachimiak A, Goodman SL, Arnaout MA. Crystal structure of the extracellular segment of integrin $\alpha v\beta 3$. Science. 2001;294(5541):339–345. doi:10.1126/science.1064535

[16] Wegener KL, Campbell ID. Transmembrane and cytoplasmic domains in integrin activation and protein-protein interactions. Mol Membr Biol. 2008;25(5):376–387. doi: 10.1080/09687680802269886

[17] Barczyk M, Carracedo S, Gullberg D. Integrins. Cell Tissue Res. 2010;339(1):269–280. doi:10.1007/s00441-009-0834-6

[18] Wegener KL, Partridge AW, Han J, Pickford AR, Liddington RC, Ginsberg MH, Cambell ID. Structural basis of integrin activation by talin. Cell. 2007;128(1):171–182. doi:10.1016/j.cell.2006.10.048

[19] Montanez E, Ussar S, Schifferer M, Bosl M, Zent R, Moser M, Fassler R. Kindlin-2 controls bidirectional signaling of integrins. Genes Dev. 2008;22:1325–1330. doi:10.1101/gad.469408.

[20] Zaidel-Bar R, Itzkovitz S, Ma'ayan A, Iyengar R, Geiger B. Functional atlas of the integrin adhesome. Nat Cell Biol. 2007;9:858–867. doi:10.1038/ncb0807-858

[21] Takada Y, Ye X, Simon S. The integrins. Genome Biol. 2007;8(5):215. doi:10.1186/gb-2007-8-5-215

[22] Srichai MB, Zent R. Integrin structure and function. In: Zent R, Pozzi A, editors. Cell-extracellular matrix interactions in cancer. 1st ed. New York: Springer-Verlag; 2010. p. 19–41. doi:10.1007/978-1-4419-0814-8

[23] Albelda SM, Buck CA. Integrins and other cell adhesion molecules. FASEB J. 1990;4(11): 2868–2880. doi:10.1038/346425a0

[24] Kuphal S, Bauer R, Bosserhoff A-K. Integrin signaling in malignant melanoma. Cancer Metastasis Rev. 2005;24(2):195–222. doi:10.1007/s10555-005-1572-1

[25] Mizejewski GJ. Role of integrins in cancer: survey of expression patterns. Proc Soc Exp Biol Med. 1999;222(2):124–138. doi:10.1046/j.1525-1373.1999.d01-122.x

[26] Cheresh DA. Structure, function and biological properties of integrin alpha v beta 3 on human melanoma cells. Cancer Metastasis Rev. 1991;10(1):3–10. doi:10.1007/BF00046839

[27] Kramer RH, Vu M, Cheng YF, Ramos DM. Integrin expression in malignant melanoma. Cancer Metastasis Rev. 1991;10(1):49–59. doi:10.1007/BF00046843

[28] Felding-Habermann B. Integrin adhesion receptors in tumor metastasis. Clin Exp Metastasis. 2003;20(3):203–213. doi:10.1023/A:1022983000355

[29] Laidler P, Gil D, Pituch-Noworolska A, Ciołczyk D, Ksiazek D, Przybyło M, Lityńska A. Expression of beta1-integrins and N-cadherin in bladder cancer and melanoma cell lines. Acta Biochim Pol. 2000;47(4):1159–1170.

[30] Qian F, Zhang ZC, Wu XF, Li YP, Xu Q. Interaction between integrin alpha(5) and fibronectin is required for metastasis of B16F10 melanoma cells. Biochem Biophys Res Commun. 2005;333(4):1269–1275. doi:10.1016/j.bbrc.2005.06.039

[31] Natali PG, Nicotra MR, Bartolazzi A, Cavaliere R, Bigotti A. Integrin expression in cutaneous malignant melanoma: association of the alpha 3/beta 1 heterodimer with tumor progression. Int J Cancer. 1993;54(1):68–72. doi:10.1002/ijc.2910540112

[32] Gehlsen KR, Davis GE, Sriramarao P. Integrin expression in human melanoma cells with differing invasive and metastatic properties. Clin Exp Metastasis. 1992;10(2):111–120. doi:10.1007/BF00114587

[33] Voura EB, Ramjeesingh RA, Montgomery AM, Siu CH. Involvement of integrin alpha(v)beta(3) and cell adhesion molecule L1 in transendothelial migration of melanoma cells. Mol Biol Cell. 2001;12(9):2699–2710. doi:10.1091/mbc.12.9.2699

[34] Albelda SM, Mette SA, Elder DE, Stewart R, Damjanovich L, Herlyn M, Buck CA. Integrin distribution in malignant melanoma: association of the beta 3 subunit with tumor progression. Cancer Res. 1990;50(20):6757–6764.

[35] Koistinen P, Ahonen M, Kähäri VM, Heino J. alphaV integrin promotes *in vitro* and *in vivo* survival of cells in metastatic melanoma. Int J Cancer. 2004;112(1):61–70. doi:10.1002/ijc.20377

[36] Ochwat D, Hoja-łukowicz D, Lityńska A. N-glycoproteins bearing β1–6 branched oligosaccharides from the A375 human melanoma cell line analysed by tandem mass spectrometry. Melanoma Res. 2004;14(6):479–485.

[37] Przybyło M, Martuszewska D, Pocheć E, Hoja-łukowicz D, Lityńska A. Identification of proteins bearing β1–6 branched N-glycans in human melanoma cell lines from different progression stages by tandem mass spectrometry analysis. Biochim Biophys Acta. 2007;1770(9):1427–1435. doi:10.1016/j.bbagen.2007.05.006

[38] Neto DS, Pantaleão L, de Sα BC, Landman G. Alpha-v-beta3 integrin expression in melanocytic nevi and cutaneous melanoma. J Cutan Pathol. 2007;34(11):851–856. doi:10.1111/j.1600-0560.2007.00730.x

[39] Ziober BL, Chen YQ, Ramos DM, Waleh N, Kramer RH. Expression of the alpha7beta1 laminin receptor suppresses melanoma growth and metastatic potential. Cell Growth Differ. 1999;10(7):479–490.

[40] Danen EHJ. Integrin signaling as a cancer drug target. ISRN Cell Biol. 2013;Article ID 135164, doi:10.1155/2013/135164

[41] Frisch SM, Ruoslahti E. Integrins and anoikis. Curr Opin Cell Biol. 1997;9(5):701–706. doi:10.1016/S0955-0674(97)80124-X

[42] van der Flier A, Sonnenberg A. Function and interactions of integrins. Cell Tissue Res. 2001;305(3):285–298. doi:10.1007/s004410100417

[43] Watt FM. Role of integrins in regulating epidermal adhesion, growth and differentiation. EMBO J. 2002;21(15):3919–3926. doi:10.1093/emboj/cdf399

[44] Rathinam R, Alahari SK. Important role of integrins in the cancer biology. Cancer Metastasis Rev. 2010;9(1):2232–2237. doi:10.1007/s10555-010-9211-x

[45] Yamada KM, Even-Ram S. Integrin regulation of growth factor receptors. Nat Cell Biol. 2002;4(4):E75–E76. doi:10.1038/ncb0402-e75

[46] Hehlgans S, Haase M, Cordes N. Signalling via integrins: implications for cell survival and anticancer strategies. Biochim Biophys Acta. 2007;1775(1):163–180. doi:10.1016/j.bbcan.2006.09.001

[47] Harburger DS, Calderwood DA. Integrin signalling at a glance. J Cell Sci. 2009;122(Pt 2):159–163. doi:10.1242/jcs.018093

[48] Christiansen MN, Chik J, Lee L, Anugraham M, Abrahams JL, Packer NH. Cell surface protein glycosylation in cancer. Proteomics. 2014;14(4–5):525–546. doi:10.1002/pmic.201300387

[49] Schadendorf D, Gawlik C, Haney U, Ostmeier H, Suter L, Czarnetzki BM. Tumour progression and metastatic behaviour *in vivo* correlates with integrin expression on melanocytic tumours. J Pathol. 1993;170(4):429–434. doi:10.1002/path.1711700405

[50] Guo W, Giancotti FG. Integrin signalling during tumour progression. Nat Rev Mol Cell Biol. 2004;5(10):816–826. doi:10.1038/nrm1490

[51] Danen EHJ. Integrins: regulators of tissue function and cancer progression. Curr Pharm Des. 2005;11(7):881–891. doi:10.2174/1381612053381756

[52] Ganguly KK, Pal S, Moulik S, Chatterjee A. Integrins and metastasis. Cell Adh Migr. 2013;7(3):251–261. doi:10.4161/cam.23840

[53] Seguin L, Desgrosellier JS, Weis SM, Cheresh DA. Integrins and cancer: regulators of cancer stemness, metastasis, and drug resistance. Trends Cell Biol. 2015;25(4):234–240. doi:10.1016/j.tcb.2014.12.006

[54] Janik ME, Lityńska A, Vereecken P. Cell migration—the role of integrin glycosylation. Biochim Biophys Acta. 2010;1800(6):545–555. doi:10.1016/j.bbagen.2010.03.013

[55] Yuan Y, Wu L, Shen S, Wu S, Burdick MM. Effect of alpha 2,6 sialylation on integrin-mediated adhesion of breast cancer cells to fibronectin and collagen IV. Life Sci. 2016;149:138–145. doi:10.1016/j.lfs.2016.02.071

[56] Gu J, Taniguchi N. Regulation of integrin functions by N-glycans. Glycoconj J. 2004;21(1–2):9–15. doi:10.1023/B:GLYC.0000043741.47559.30

[57] Pigott R, Power C. The adhesion molecules facts book. 1st ed. London: Academic Press; 1993.

[58] Pocheć E, Lityńska A, Amoresano A, Casbarra A. Glycosylation profile of integrin alpha 3 beta 1 changes with melanoma progression. Biochim Biophys Acta. 2003;1643(1–3): 113–123. doi:10.1016/j.bbamcr.2003.10.004

[59] Pocheć E, Bubka M, Rydlewska M, Janik M, Pokrywka M, Lityńska A. Aberrant glycosylation of $\alpha v \beta 3$ integrin is associated with melanoma progression. Anticancer Res. 2015;5(4):2093–2103.

[60] Veiga SS, Chammas R, Cella N, Brentani RR. Glycosylation of beta-1 integrins in B16-F10 mouse melanoma cells as determinant of differential binding and acquisition of biological activity. Int J Cancer. 1995;61(3):420–424. doi:10.1002/ijc.2910610324

[61] Fuster MM, Esko JD. The sweet and sour of cancer: glycans as novel therapeutic targets. Nat Rev Cancer. 2005;5(7):526–542. doi:10.1038/nrc1649

[62] Stanley P, Schachter H, Taniguchi N. N-gycans. In: Varki A, Cummings RD, Esko JD, Freeze HH, Stanley P, Bertozzi CR, Hart GW, Etzler ME, editors. Essentials of glycobiology. 2nd ed. Cold Spring Harbor, NY: Cold Spring Harbor Laboratory Press; 2009.

[63] Spiro RC, Laufer DM, Perry SK, Harper JR. Effect of inhibitors of N-linked oligosaccharide processing on the cell surface expression of a melanoma integrin. J Cell Biochem. 1989;41(1):37–45. doi:10.1002/jcb.240410105

[64] Zheng M, Fang H, Hakomori S. Functional role of N-glycosylation in alpha 5 beta 1 integrin receptor. De-N-glycosylation induces dissociation or altered association of alpha 5 and beta 1 subunits and concomitant loss of fibronectin binding activity. J Biol Chem. 1994;269(16):12325–12331.

[65] Isaji T, Sato Y, Fukuda T, Gu J. N-glycosylation of the I-like domain of $\beta 1$ integrin domain is essential for $\beta 1$ integrin expression and biological function. J Biol Chem. 2009;284(18);12207–12216. doi:10.1074/jbc.M807920200

[66] Chammas R, Veiga SS, Line S, Potocnjak P, Brentani RR. Asn-linked oligosaccharide-dependent interaction between laminin and gp120/140. An alpha 6/beta 1 integrin. J Biol Chem. 1991;266(5):3349–3355.

[67] Chammas R, Veiga SS, Travassos LR, Brentani RR. Functionally distinct roles for glycosylation of alpha and beta integrin chains in cell-matrix interactions. Proc Natl Acad Sci U S A. 1993;90(5):1795–1799. doi:10.1073/pnas.90.5.1795

[68] Bironaite D, Nesland JM, Dalen H, Risberg B, Bryne M. N-Glycans influence the *in vitro* adhesive and invasive behaviour of three metastatic cell lines. Tumour Biol. 2000;21(3): 165–175. doi:10.1159/000030123

[69] Passaniti A, Hart GW. Cell surface sialylation and tumor metastasis. Metastatic potential of B16 melanoma variants correlates with their relative numbers of specific penultimate oligosaccharide structures. J Biol Chem. 1988;263(16):7591–7603.

[70] Chammas R, Veiga SS, Brentani RR. Glycobiology of laminin-integrin interaction and the metastatic phenotype. Mem Inst Oswaldo Cruz. 1991;86(Suppl 3):29–35. doi: 10.1590/S0074-02761991000700006

[71] Kawano T, Takasaki S, Tao TW, Kobata A. Altered glycosylation of beta 1 integrins associated with reduced adhesiveness to fibronectin and laminin. Int J Cancer. 1993;53(1):91–96. doi:10.1002/ijc.2910530118

[72] Ogura T, Noguchi T, Murai-Takebe R, Hosooka T, Honma N, Kasuga M. Resistance of B16 melanoma cells to CD47-induced negative regulation of motility as a result of aberrant N-glycosylation of SHPS-1. J Biol Chem. 2004;279(14):13711–13720. doi: 10.1074/jbc.M310276200

[73] Reddy BV, Kalraiya RD. Sialilated beta1,6 branched N-oligosaccharides modulate adhesion, chemotaxis and motility of melanoma cells: effect on invasion and spontaneous metastasis properties. Biochim Biophys Acta. 2006;1760(9):1393–1402. doi: 10.1016/j.bbagen.2006.05.003

[74] Pocheć E, Janik M, Hoja-łukowicz D, Link-Lenczowski P, Przybyło M, Lityńska A. Expression of integrins $\alpha3\beta1$ and $\alpha5\beta1$ and GlcNAc $\beta1,6$ glycan branching influences metastatic melanoma cell migration on fibronectin. Eur J Cell Biol. 2013;92(12):355–362. doi:10.1016/j.ejcb.2013.10.007

[75] Kremser ME, Przybyło M, Hoja-łukowicz D, Pocheć E, Amoresano A, Carpentieri A, Bubka M, Lityńska A. Characterisation of alpha3beta1 and alpha(v)beta3 integrin N-oligosaccharides in metastatic melanoma WM9 and WM239 cell lines. Biochim Biophys Acta. 2008;1780(12):1421–1431. doi:10.1016/j.bbagen.2008.07.011

[76] Janik ME, Przybyło M, Pocheć E, Pokrywka M, Lityńska A. Effect of $\alpha3\beta1$ and $\alpha v\beta3$ integrin glycosylation on interaction of melanoma cells with vitronectin. Acta Biochim Pol. 2010;57(1):55–61.

[77] Dennis JW, Laferté S, Waghorne C, Breitman ML, Kerbel RS. Beta 1-6 branching of Asn-linked oligosaccharides is directly associated with metastasis. Science. 1987;236(4801): 582–585. doi:10.1126/science.2953071

[78] Taniguchi N, Miyoshi E, Ko JH, Ikeda Y, Ihara Y. Implication of N-acetylglucosaminyltransferases III and V in cancer: gene regulation and signaling mechanism. Biochim Biophys Acta. 1999;1455(2–3):287–300. doi:10.1016/S0925-4439(99)00066-6

[79] Couldrey C, Green JE. Metastases: the glycan connection. Breast Cancer Res. 2000;2(5): 321–323. doi:10.1186/bcr75

[80] Guo HB, Lee I, Kamar M, Akiyama SK, Pierce M. Aberrant N-glycosylation of beta1 integrin causes reduced alpha5beta1 integrin clustering and stimulates cell migration. Cancer Res. 2002;62(23):6837–6845.

[81] Wang L, Liang Y, Li Z, Cai X, Zhang W, Wu G, Jin J, Fang Z, Yang Y, Zha X. Increase in beta1-6 GlcNAc branching caused by N-acetylglucosaminyltransferase V directs

integrin beta1 stability in human hepatocellular carcinoma cell line SMMC-7721. J Cell Biochem. 2007;100(1):230–241. doi:10.1002/jcb.21071

[82] Yagel S, Feinmesser R, Waghorne C, Lala PK, Breitman ML, Dennis JW. Evidence that beta 1-6 branched Asn-linked oligosaccharides on metastatic tumor cells facilitate invasion of basement membranes. Int J Cancer. 1989;44(4):685–690. doi:10.1002/ijc.2910440422

[83] Dennis JW, Granovsky M, Warren CE. Glycoprotein glycosylation and cancer progression. Biochim Biophys Acta. 1999;1473(1):21–34. doi:10.1016/S0304-4165(99)00167-1

[84] Ranjan A, Kalraiya RD. Invasive potential of melanoma cells correlates with the expression of MT1-MMP and regulated by modulating its association with motility receptors via N-glycosylation on the receptors. Biomed Res Int. 2014;2014:804680. doi:10.1155/2014/804680

[85] Ranjan A, Bane SM, Kalraiya RD. Glycosylation of the laminin receptor (α3β1) regulates its association with tetraspanin CD151: impact on cell spreading, motility, degradation and invasion of basement membrane by tumor cells. Exp Cell Res. 2014;322(2):249–264. doi:10.1016/j.yexcr.2014.02.004

[86] Baldwin G, Novitskaya V, Sadej R, Pochec E, Litynska A, Hartmann C, Williams J, Ashman L, Eble JA, Berditchevski F. Tetraspanin CD151 regulates glycosylation of (alpha)3(beta)1 integrin. J Biol Chem. 2008;283(51):35445–35454. doi:10.1074/jbc.M806394200

[87] Pocheć E, Ząbczyńska M, Bubka M, Homa J, Lityńska A. β1,6-branched complex-type N-glycans affect FAK signaling in metastatic melanoma cells. Cancer Invest. 2016;34(1):45–56. doi:10.3109/07357907.2015.1102928

[88] Tsuji T, Kawada Y, Kai-Murozono M, Komatsu S, Han SA, Takeuchi K, Mizushima H, Miyazaki K, Irimura T. Regulation of melanoma cell migration and invasion by laminin-5 and alpha3beta1 integrin (VLA-3). Clin Exp Metastasis. 2002;19(2):127–134. doi:10.1023/A:1014573204062

[89] Giannelli G, Astigiano S, Antonaci S, Morini M, Barbieri O, Noonan DM, Albini A. Role of the alpha3beta1 and alpha6beta4 integrins in tumor invasion. Clin Exp Metastasis. 2002;19(3):217–223. doi:10.1023/A:1015579204607

[90] Litynska A, Przybylo M, Pochec E, Kremser E, Hoja-Lukowicz D, Sulowska U. Does glycosylation of melanoma cells influence their interactions with fibronectin? Biochimie. 2006;88(5):527–534. doi:10.1016/j.biochi.2005.10.012

[91] Melchiori A, Mortarini R, Carlone S, Marchisio PC, Anichini A, Noonan DM, Albini A. The alpha 3 beta 1 integrin is involved in melanoma cell migration and invasion. Exp Cell Res. 1995;219(1):233–242. doi:10.1006/excr.1995.1223

[92] Kreidberg JA. Functions of alpha3beta1 integrin. Curr Opin Cell Biol. 2000;12(5):548–553. doi:10.1016/S0955-0674(00)00130-7

[93] Prokopishyn NL, Puzon-McLaughlin W, Takada Y, Laferté S. Integrin alpha3beta1 expressed by human colon cancer cells is a major carrier of oncodevelopmental carbohydrate epitopes. J Cell Biochem. 1999;72(2):189–209. doi:10.1002/(SICI)1097-4644(19990201)72:2<189::AID-JCB4>3.0.CO;2-N

[94] Link-Lenczowski P, Butters TD, Litynska A. Glycosylation profile of integrin alpha3beta1 subunits in human melanoma cells at different stages of progression. In: XXI International Symposium on Glycoconjugates (GLYCO 21); 21–26 August. 2011; Vienna. Austria: Glycoconjugate J; 2011. p. 329.

[95] Béliveau A, Bérubé M, Rousseau A, Pelletier G, Guérin SL. Expression of integrin alpha5beta1 and MMPs associated with epithelioid morphology and malignancy of uveal melanoma. Invest Ophthalmol Vis Sci. 2000;41(8):2363–2372.

[96] Schaffner F, Ray AM, Dontenwill M. Integrin $\alpha5\beta1$, the fibronectin receptor, as a pertinent therapeutic target in solid tumors. Cancers. 2013;5(1):27–47. doi:10.3390/cancers5010027

[97] Ruoslahti E. The Walter Herbert Lecture. Control of cell motility and tumour invasion by extracellular matrix interactions. Br J Cancer. 1992;66(2):239–242. doi:10.1038/bjc.1992.250

[98] Aznavoorian S, Stracke ML, Parsons J, McClanahan J, Liotta LA. Integrin alphavbeta3 mediates chemotactic and haptotactic motility in human melanoma cells through different signaling pathways. J Biol Chem. 1996;271(6):3247–3254. doi:10.1074/jbc.271.6.3247

[99] Zhao Y, Nakagawa T, Itoh S, Inamori K, Isaji T, Kariya Y, Kondo A, Miyoshi E, Miyazaki K, Kawasaki N, Taniguchi N, Gu J. N-acetylglucosaminyltransferase III antagonizes the effect of N-acetylglucosaminyltransferase V on alpha3beta1 integrin-mediated cell migration. J Biol Chem. 2006;281(43):32122–32130. doi:10.1074/jbc.M607274200

[100] Friedl P, Wolf K. Tumour-cell invasion and migration: diversity and escape mechanisms. Nat Rev Cancer. 2003;3(5):362–374. doi:10.1038/nrm2720

[101] Przybyło M, Pocheć E, Link-Lenczowski P, Lityńska A. Beta1-6 branching of cell surface glycoproteins may contribute to uveal melanoma progression by up-regulating cell motility. Mol Vis. 2008;14:625–636.

[102] Akiyama SK. Integrins in cell adhesion and signaling. Hum Cell. 1996;9(3):181–186.

[103] Zhao Y, Sato Y, Isaji T, Fukuda T, Matsumoto A, Miyoshi E, Gu J, Taniguchi N. Branched N-glycans regulate the biological functions of integrins and cadherins. FEBS J. 2008;275(9):1939–1948. doi:10.1111/j.1742-4658.2008.06346.x

[104] Gu J, Sato Y, Kariya Y, Isaji T, Taniguchi N, Fukuda T. A mutual regulation between cell-cell adhesion and N-glycosylation: implication of the bisecting GlcNAc for biological functions. J Proteome Res. 2009;8(2):431–435. doi:10.1021/pr800674g

[105] Kugler MC, Wei Y, Chapman HA. Urokinase receptor and integrin interactions. Curr Pharm Des. 2003;9(19):1565–1574. doi:10.2174/1381612033454658

[106] Stahl A, Mueller BM. Binding of urokinase to its receptor promotes migration and invasion of human melanoma cells *in vitro*. Cancer Res. 1994;54(11):3066–3071.

[107] Laurenzana A, Biagioni A, D'Alessio S, Bianchini F, Chillŕ A, Margheri F, Luciani C, Mazzanti B, Pimpinelli N, Torre E, Danese S, Calorini L, Del Rosso M, Fibbi G. Melanoma cell therapy: endothelial progenitor cells as shuttle of the MMP12 uPAR-degrading enzyme. Oncotarget. 2014;5(11):3711–3727. doi:10.18632/oncotarget.1987

[108] Varki A. Sialic acids as ligands in recognition phenomena. FASEB J. 1997;11(4):248–255.

[109] Traving C, Schauer R. Structure, function and metabolism of sialic acids. Cell Mol Life Sci. 1998;54(12):1330–1349. doi:10.1007/s000180050258

[110] Schultz MJ, Swindall AF, Bellis SL. Regulation of the metastatic cell phenotype by sialylated glycans. Cancer Metastasis Rev. 2012;31(3–4):501–518. doi:10.1007/s10555-012-9359-7

[111] Yogeeswaran G, Salk PL. Metastatic potential is positively correlated with cell surface sialylation of cultured murine tumor cell lines. Science. 1981;212(4502):1514–1516. doi:10.1126/science.7233237

[112] Sato T. Lectin-probed western blot analysis. Methods Mol Biol. 2014;1200:93–100. doi:10.1007/978-1-4939-1292-6_8

[113] Ranjan A, Kalraiya RD. α2,6 sialylation associated with increased beta 1,6-branched N-oligosaccharides influences cellular adhesion and invasion. J Biosci. 2013;38(5):867–876. doi:10.1007/s12038-013-9382-z

[114] Chang WW, Yu CY, Lin TW, Wang PH, Tsai YC. Soyasaponin I decreases the expression of alpha2,3-linked sialic acid on the cell surface and suppresses the metastatic potential of B16F10 melanoma cells. Biochem Biophys Res Commun. 2006;341(2):614–619. doi:10.1016/j.bbrc.2005.12.216

[115] Nadanaka S, Sato C, Kitajima K, Katagiri K, Irie S, Yamagata T. Occurrence of oligosialic acids on integrin alpha 5 subunit and their involvement in cell adhesion to fibronectin. J Biol Chem. 2001;276(36):33657–33664. doi:10.1074/jbc.M011100200

Chapter 4

Bitter Sweetness of Malignant Melanoma: Deciphering the Role of Cell Surface Glycosylation in Tumour Progression and Metastasis

Małgorzata Przybyło, Marcelina E. Janik and Dorota Hoja-Łukowicz

Additional information is available at the end of the chapter

http://dx.doi.org/10.5772/64406

Abstract

Malignant melanoma is the sixth most commonly diagnosed cancer in developed countries. Like in many cancers, survival rates are closely associated with the time of melanoma detection. Regrettably, most cases of melanoma are caught at diffuse state and methods used in clinical practice and experimental trials are not effective. Thus, there is a great interest in discovering biomarkers that could be used for screening those with melanoma, as prognostic and prediction factors as well as new potential targets for melanoma treatment. For this purpose, many groups have examined alteration in the structure and expression of carbohydrate part of glycoconjugates to identify changes that occur with melanoma. The observed changes include increased β1,6 branching correlating with higher abundance of polylactosamine extension, increased sialylation accompanied by differences in the position of sialic acid residues, increased fucosylation, higher levels of T and Tn antigens as well as changes in the expression of ganglioside structures. As a consequence of glycan modification, the loosened matrix adhesion, increased motility, higher invasive potential and metastasis formation have been observed. Growth and migration of melanoma cells have been also found to be stimulated by advanced glycation end products. Biomarker discovery is a multi-step process and the recent glycomic data on melanoma are mostly related to the discovery phase, as the first one leading to validation and standardisation steps.

Keywords: glycosylation, glycation, malignant melanoma, tumour-associated carbohydrate antigens

1. Introduction

The population of patients with cutaneous melanoma is one of the most rapidly increasing cancer groups worldwide over the last 50 years in most fair-skinned populations [1, 2]. The vast majority of cases (almost 85%) occur in developed countries, where melanoma is the sixth most commonly diagnosed cancer. Despite the improvements in the diagnosis thereof, the best chance of melanoma recovery remains the surgical removal of a thin early-stage lesion, because methods used on large scale in clinical practices as well as experimental trials are not able to cure this type of cancer at diffuse state [3, 4]. Palliative treatment for inoperable recurrence or metastatic disease is frequently toxic and ineffective. Thus, appropriate means for predicting prognosis or effective treatments are still needed.

Understanding the biology of tumour cells is an important factor for the development of new strategies for cancer treatment. Unfortunately, reliable biomarkers are not available for the vast majority of cancers. Macro-molecules present at the cell membrane surface and in the membranes themselves constitute an important field for study in the understanding of cancer cell behaviour. Nowadays, investigation on structural properties and function of cancer-associated glycosylation changes, as indicators of tumourigenesis, is gaining more attention in order to discover new markers suitable for early detection, for differentiating between benign and malignant stages and for therapeutic purposes. For a long time carbohydrates have been merely regarded as an integral structural component of glycoconjugates (glycoproteins, glycolipids and proteoglycans) and a storage material. Although they are ubiquitous constituents of almost all living organisms, glycoconjugates were believed to be deprived of any biological function. Progress in glycoconjugates research due to application of new powerful tools has enabled researches to discover the broad range of biological activities in which carbohydrates are involved [5–8]. Glycoconjugates participate in several processes, including protein conformational stability, protection from proteolytic degradation, protein thermal stability, biological activity, protein targeting, circulating life-time and their ultimate fate, immunogenicity, the transduction of information between cells, sperm-egg interactions, leukocyte traffic to sites of inflammation, leukocyte migration (homing) to lymphoid organs, blood clotting, apoptosis and host-pathogen interactions. Moreover, changes in glycoconjugates have been proved to be associated with a number of pathological processes, for example, carbohydrate deficiency diseases, inflammation, allergy, rheumatoid arthritis, thrombosis, infarction, diabetes and cancer [7, 9–12]. The aim of this chapter is to highlight the contribution of the defined tumour-associated carbohydrate antigens present on the cell surface of melanoma cells to their behaviour during tumour progression and metastasis, as well as to present glycomic opportunities in defining markers for melanoma early detection, disease progression or predicting therapy outcome that might help to defeat one of the deadliest forms of cancer.

2. Glycoconjugates and cancer

Glycosylation is the most frequent post-translational modification of macro-molecules. Carbohydrate part (glycan) biosynthesis involves various types of glycosyltransferases, glycosidases and sugar nucleotides [8, 13]. As glycosylation is not template-driven, but is indirectly controlled by a number of genes (1–2% of translated genome) and the environmental factors integrate at the level of glycan biosynthesis, the relative amounts and structure of glycans is cell-, tissue- and species-dependent [14]. The biosynthetic basis of such diversity consists in the alteration in the activity of various glycosyltransferases and competition between enzymes for acceptor intermediates during glycan elongation. Additionally, in cancer cells the activity of glycosyltransferases and glycosidases is controlled by other factors such as the levels of nucleotide sugars and their transporters, the expression of chaperons that regulate protein folding and quality control of proteins, endogenous lectin as well as by altered expression of the enzymes engaged in biosynthetic process together with their proper localisation [15]. Recently, it has been shown that the aberrant expression of glyco-genes in cancer is also due to aberrant promotor methylation. In melanoma a difference in methylation of 20 genes involved in O-glycosylation has been stated [16]. These results suggest new potential targets for melanoma treatment, and indicate that the methylation status of selected glyco-genes might be used for prognostic purposes.

The hallmarks of all types of human, as well as experimental rodent cancers include profound changes in the structure and expression of carbohydrate part of glycoconjugates, resulting from activation of particular oncogenes or rearrangements of glycan biosynthetic pathways [1, 11, 12, 17]. Generally, cancer-associated changes in glycosylation profile are associated either with the expression and secretion of inappropriate glycosylated molecules or the appearance of new antigens (onco-foetal or *de novo* synthesised antigens). Some of the cancer-associated carbohydrate antigens have found their clinical application as a target for the diagnosis of different types of tumours (breast, ovarian and prostate cancers) or as therapeutic agents (glycoconjugate vaccines) [7, 9, 11, 12, 18–26]. Interestingly, among at least 100 cancer biomarkers used currently for the diagnosis of different types of tumours, the vast majority includes glycoproteins and glycolipids, and they are measured immunochemically using monoclonal antibodies [27]. However, these monoclonal antibodies against glycoprotein are in most cases aimed not towards the glycan epitope, but towards the protein chain. The most frequently observed changes in glycosylation structure during malignant transformation are the extensive expression of β1,6-branched N-glycans, the increased expression of bisected N-glycans, increased cell surface sialylation frequently accompanied by differences in the position of sialic acid residues including the expression of onco-foetal α-2,8-linked polysialic acid, the expression of core fucosylated and non-fucosylated paucimannose-type structures, premature termination of O-glycan biosynthesis in mucins leading to the presence of the so-called pan-tumour antigens, i.e. T (Galβ1–3GalNAc-α1-O-Ser/Thr), Tn (GalNAc-α1-O-Ser/Thr) and sialyl-Tn (Siaα2-6GalNAc-α1-O-Ser/Thr) mucin antigens, abnormalities in the expression of ABO blood group and tissue antigens [15].

Protein-carbohydrate interactions have not only biological but also medical implication, since glycosylation profile is dynamically modified by many intra- and/or extra-cellular stimuli. Additionally, these interactions are involved in the control of cell homeostasis and its social behaviour. Therefore, alterations in carbohydrate structures of glycoconjugates including cell adhesion molecules, commonly found in various tumours, are considered to be the basis for abnormal social behaviour of tumour cells, such as invasion to the surrounding tissue and metastasis, loose of cell-cell contact and epithelial-mesenchymal transition (EMT) [15, 18, 28–34]. These macro-molecules could also significantly change antigenicity and immunogenicity of tumour cells and therefore promote tumour progression by chronic inflammation and angiogenesis [24].

3. Glycosylation and melanoma

Over 5000 cell lines are currently available for studying cutaneous and ocular melanoma, which covers different stages of the disease progression from primary melanomas to metastases in distinct organs [35]. The most frequently used model to study the linkage between glycosylation and metastatic behaviour of melanoma cells is B16 murine melanoma cell line and its sub-lines of a different metastatic potential. Detailed analysis of B16 sub-lines with high- and low-metastatic potentials has revealed that although these sub-lines expressed comparable amount of sialic acids, α2,3-linked sialic acids were predominantly found in high-metastatic sub-line, while α2,6-linked sialic acids were observed in low-metastatic sub-line [36]. Other studies performed on a poorly metastasising wheat germ agglutinin-resistant mutants of B16 melanoma cells have proved that the variant cell line displayed well-defined changes in its cell surface glycosylation profile in comparison to wild-type cells, involving the decrease in the number of side chains in oligosaccharides, the loss of sialic acids α2,3-linked to galactose, concomitant with the increase in the amount of fucose α1,3-linked to N-acetylglucosamine [37]. Such cells were less adherent to extracellular matrix components and showed decreased metastatic potential. The observed effects resulted from a 60-fold increase in α1,3-fucosyltransferase activity, while sialyltransferase activity did not decrease significantly [38]. Participation of sialic acids in metastasis formation has been also demonstrated by transfection of murine B16, JB/RH and JB/MS cells with gene for α1,3-galactosyltransferase (α1,3GT). α1,3GT competes with α2,3-sialyltransferase and α2,6-sialyltransferase for the same acceptor, i.e. N-acetyllactosamine moieties (**Figure 1**) [39]. The transfected cells showed reduced metastasis formation which was caused by the reduction of cell membrane sialylation. Similar great reduction of metastatic capacity has been observed after the use of swainsonine (SW), a competitive inhibitor of Golgi α-mannosidase II which stops N-oligosaccharide synthesis on hybrid and high-mannose-type structures preventing the synthesis of complex-type structures (**Figure 1**) [40]. It has also been demonstrated that the loss of sialylated lactosamine antenae and decreased branching of N-oligosaccharides on B16-F10 melanoma cells (cells of high incidence of lung colonisation) reduced their pulmonary colonisation when the cells were injected into the circulation of syngeneic mice [41]. This was consistent with the observation that SW treatment of athymic nude mice bearing human MeWo cells significantly reduced solid tumour growth and inhibited tumour cell proliferation both *in vitro* and *in vivo* [42]. Interestingly, SW has been reported to show evidence of clinical efficacy in a phase I clinical trial [43]. Metastatic capacities of highly metastatic B16-hm melanoma cells have also been down-regulated by introduction of β1,4-N-acetylglucosaminyltransferase III (GnT-III) gene, which codes the enzyme that catalyses the formation of bisecting N-acetylglucosamine in N-oligosaccharide chains [44]. One of the targets of GnT-III in the transfected cells was E-cadherin. GnT-III gene transfected cells showed increased E-cadherin-dependent cell-cell adhesion and suppression of lung metastasis formation as well as decreased level of cell adhesion to laminin and collagen [44, 45]. Taken together, these results strongly suggested that highly branched and sialylated N-oligosaccharides present on cell surface glycoconjugates contribute to effective melanoma cell metastasis. Interestingly, N-glycosylation in human melanoma SK-MEL-2 cells has also been found to play an important role in maintenance of viability thereof through the regulation of insulin-like growth factor-1 receptor translocation to the cell surface [46, 47].

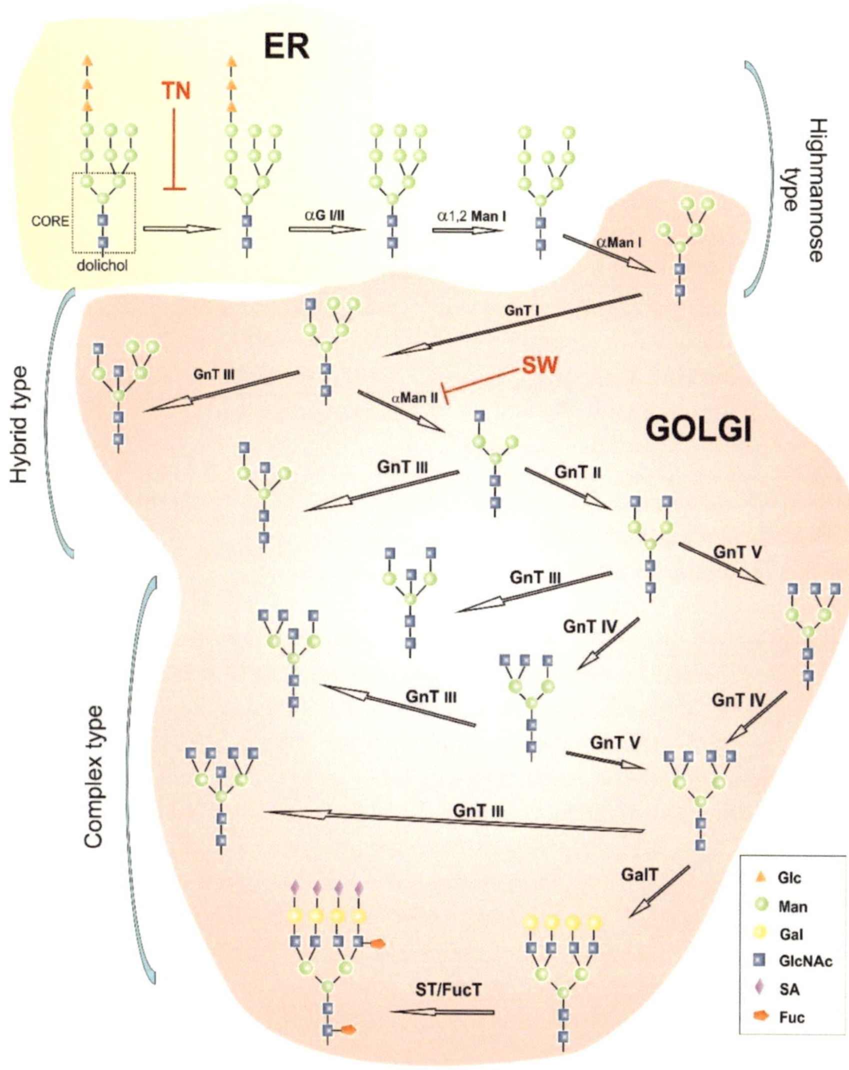

Figure 1. Structures and synthetic pathway of N-oligosaccharides.

β1,6-Branched N-oligosaccharides are tri- and tetra-antennary complex-type N-glycans formed due to the action of N-acetylglucosaminyltransferase V (GnT-V), which catalyses the transfer of GlcNAc from UDP-GlcNAc to the 6-OH position of α-Man residue in α6 arm (**Figure 1**). In malignant transformation, the increased β1,6-branching is a result of enhanced activity of GnT-V associated with the increased expression of GnT-V gene (i.e. *Mgat5*), which is in turn regulated by Ras/Raf/MAPK, a signalling pathway commonly activated in tumour cells, and the Ets family including Ets-1 transcription factor [48, 49]. Ets-1 transcription factor, in turn, is known to regulate several molecules associated with cell invasiveness and metastasis, such as cyclin D (cell-cycle progression), vascular endothelial growth factor and basic fibroblast growth factor (potent angiogenic factors), Rho/Cdc42/rac-1 (motility) as well as matrix metalloproteinases-2, -3 and -9 (tissue remodelling) [50]. Artificial and spontaneous melanoma hybrids of high-metastatic potential have been proved to possess enhanced expression of GnT-V gene (*Mgat5*), increasing enzymatic activity of encoded glycosyltransferase [51]. Primary tumours are often infiltrated by macrophages and lymphocytes. The increased GnT-V activity and growing amount of β1,6-branched N-oligosaccharides in melanoma cells could reflect previous fusion of tumour-associated macrophages with cells of the primary tumour [52, 53]. Indeed, it has been shown that macrophage × Cloudman S91 mouse melanoma hybrids displayed increased motility *in vitro* and enhanced metastatic potential *in vivo* as well as up-regulated GnT-V activity and increased content of β1,6-branched N-glycans [51]. In macrophage-melanoma cell fusion hybrids β1,6-branched N-oligosaccharides have also been shown to be associated with enhanced melanin production and autophagy [54, 55]. A study using GnT-V knockout mice has demonstrated that although *Mgat5* products were not essential for embryonic development, when expressed in cancer cells they directly promoted tumour growth and metastasis [56].

β1,6-Branched N-oligosaccharides have been shown not to be synthesised by melanocytes or by cells of early melanoma *in situ*, but these structures are frequently found in a fully developed form of melanoma *in situ* as well as invasive and metastatic melanoma [55]. Our group, by a comparative analysis of glycoprotein pattern in four human cell line stages (primary site—WM35 cells; metastatic sites—WM9, WM239 and A375) with the use of lectins has revealed that melanoma cell lines from metastatic sites possessed more proteins being carriers of β1,6-branched N-oligosaccharides as well as α2,3- and α 2,6-linked sialic acids than those from melanoma *in situ*, as revealed by staining with *Phaseolus vulgaris* (PHAL), *Maackia amurensis* and *Sambucus nigra* agglutinins, respectively [57]. Not only the amount of β1,6-branched N-oligosaccharides progressively increased with disease progression, but also additional bands within the range of 100–160 kDa were observed by staining with PHAL. The minor differences in high-mannose-type glycan composition have also been observed in the above-mentioned four melanoma cell lines [57]. The functional importance of these type of oligosaccharides in tumourigenesis is still being studied; however, it has been shown that enhanced expression of high-mannose-type glycans on B16 murine melanoma cells promoted liver metastasis formation via mannose receptor-mediated melanoma cell attachment to hepatic sinusoidal endothelium [58]. Our further studies carried out on over 100 melanoma cell lines deposited in ESTDAB melanoma Cell Bank (Tubingen, Germany) have shown that the average number of proteins bearing β1,6-branched N-oligosaccharides was similar in uveal as well as primary and metastatic cutaneous melanoma cell lines [59]. Additionally, the expression of *Mgat5* was stated to be generally at low level; however, in 10% of cells its expression was high, while it was absent in only one cell line [59]. Comparative research on cancer-related N-glycan alteration in human melanoma WM793 cell line, which originated from early vertical growth phase lesions, and in its metastatic counterpart WM1205Lu cell line, from metastasis site in the mouse lung, has demonstrated that *Mgat-5* expression and the amount of β1,6-branched N-glycans increased with acquisition of a metastatic phenotype by melanoma cells [60]. In human melanoma biopsies, primary tumours showed heterogeneous staining for β1,6-branched N-glycans while metastases were much more homogeneous [61], suggesting that the presence of these glycans in primary tumours might be a sign of the increased metastatic competence.

It is well documented in the literature that elevated level of β1,6-branched N-oligosaccharides correlates with higher invasive potential, metastasis formation, reconstruction of the vascular system and growth of tumour cells [48]. Additionally, the loosened matrix adhesion of tumour cells may allow them to leave their original site in the tissue [62–64]. It is still a subject to identify glycoproteins bearing these structures. It is evident from the studies of our group that the expression level of β1,6-branched N-oligosaccharides is associated with acquisition of the metastatic potential in melanoma, and of particular interest are glycoproteins with the apparent molecular weight of 100–160 kDa [57]. We identified target glycoproteins of GnT-V from four human melanoma cell lines (WM35, WM9, WM239 and A375) by tandem mass spectrometry [48, 65]. Among the identified proteins, the largest group comprised integrin subunits (α2, α3, α4, α5, αv, β1 and β3). Additionally, N-cadherin, L1CAM, Mac-2 binding protein (Mac-2-BP), lysosome-associated membrane protein 1 (LAMP-1), CD44, melanoma-associated antigen (MAA), melanoma cell adhesion molecule (CD146, Mel-CAM), intracellular adhesion molecule 1 (CD54, ICAM-1), tumour rejection antigen-1 and melanoma-associated chondroitin sulphate proteoglycan 4 were found. The number of proteins being a substrate for GnT-V seemed to be better correlated with melanoma development and progression than with the expression of these cell adhesion molecules on melanoma cell surface. Independently of melanoma progression, αv and β1 integrin subunits as well as LAMP-1, CD146, CD54 and Mac-2-BP were always substrates for GnT-V; α3, α5 and β3 integrin subunits possessed no β1,6-branched N-oligosaccharides in WM35 cell line, being a radial growth phase primary melanoma, whereas α4 integrin subunit, CD44 and N-cadherin appeared to have these structures only in A375 cell line, which was the most aggressive melanoma cell line among the studied ones. It is well documented in the literature that the patterns of cell adhesion molecules differ between normal and malignant tissues. In cutaneous melanoma, the expression levels of α2β1, α3β1, α6β1 and αvβ3 integrins have been found to be associated with tumour progression. We demonstrated that not only gain or loss of adhesion molecule expression and increased level of β1,6-branched N-oligosaccharides, but also changes in the number of proteins being a substrate for GnT-V appear to be a consequence of disease progression from a tumourigenic to the metastatic phenotype. The involvement of these glycoproteins in adhesion and migration of cutaneous melanoma cells has been clearly demonstrated [60, 62, 63, 66–71]. In general, overexpression of β1,6-branched N-glycans on cell adhesion molecules contributed to the significant decrease in these cell adhesion level to extracellular matrix components, loss of contact inhibition as well as increased motility *in vitro* and enhanced metastasis *in vivo*. Similarly, the presence of α2,3- and α2,6-linked sialic acids on the cell surface has facilitated the migratory properties and enhanced invasive properties of human melanoma cells, respectively [70]. The loosened matrix adhesion of tumour cells permits them to leave their original site in the tissue. This, in turn, may facilitate the turnover of cell-cell and cell-extra-cellular matrix contacts to enhance cell motility [17, 72].

Contrary results regarding the role of β1,6-branched N-glycans were obtained when glycosylation analysis was performed on tissues isolated from patients. Studies carried out on sections of 100 primary cutaneous malignant melanoma histochemically stained with five lectins (*Sambucus nigra* agglutinin, *Phaseolus vulgaris* agglutinin, *Triticum vulgaris* agglutinin, *Maackia amurensis* agglutinin and *Helix pomatia* agglutinin) differing in their carbohydrate binding specificity, have revealed that β1,6-branched N-glycans and sialic acid residues are of no functional importance in melanoma [73], although both of them were correlated with metastasis in other malignancies (breast, lung and colon). These results obtained by Thies and colleagues [73] clearly showed that only N-acetylgalactosylamine/-glusocamine residues, recognised by *Helix pomatia* agglutinin might be linked to metastasis in human malignant melanoma. The predominant expression of Thomsen-Friedenreich (T) antigen (Galβ1-3GalNAcα1-O-Ser/Thr) versus its immature precursor (GalNAcα1-O-Ser/Thr), both of which are an uncompleted form of O-linked mucine-type glycans, has been found to be helpful in order to differentiate primary melanomas from metastatic ones [73]. The close association between Tn and sialyl-Tn antigens and neoplastic transformation prompted some researches to use them for active immunotherapy [74]. Our group has shown that nucleolin, the expression of which is positively correlated with the increased rate of cell division, was a carrier of Tn antigens and was present on the cell surface of melanoma cells [75]. As this molecule contains multiple possible MHC class I binding peptides in its sequence, it might be a target for immunodiagnostic and possibly therapeutic purposes. Interestingly, it has been found that N-glycosylation enhanced presentation of a MHC class I-restricted epitope from tyrosinase [76]. This enzyme is a membrane-associated glycoprotein and acts as antigens for immunological recognition of melanomas [77].

It has also been shown that B16 melanoma cells exhibited a fivefold higher cell surface β1,4-galactosyltransferase activity in metastatic variants than their non-metastatic counterparts [78]. This enzyme catalyses the transfer of galactose residue to terminal N-acetylglucosamine residues on the cell surface glycolipid glucosylceramide (**Figure 2**), which is a precursor of glycosphingolipids. Glycosphingolipids which possess at least one sialic acid residue constitute a broad family of molecules called gangliosides. It has been shown that gangliosides are expressed with higher abundance in tumour cells in comparison to their normal counterparts. In normal melanocytes GM3 are expressed as their major gangliosides, whereas GM3 and GD3 are synthesised predominantly in malignant melanomas [79, 80]. A few melanomas frequently synthesise small amounts of more complex gangliosides, i.e. GM2 and GD2. In human melanomas the level of GD2 expression has been found to be associated with tumour progression and metastatic potential [81].

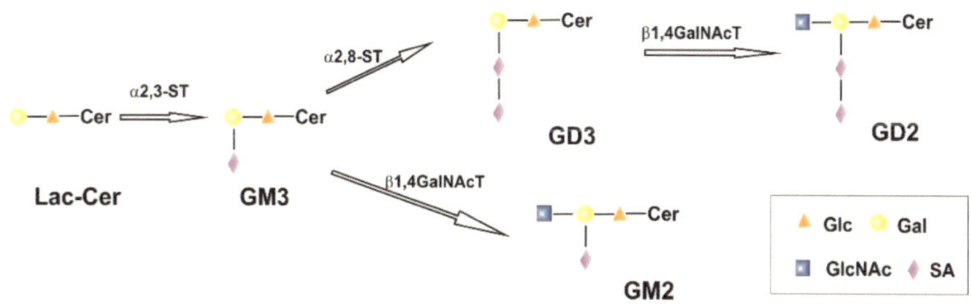

Figure 2. Structures and synthetic pathway of major gangliosides.

Ganglioside expression on individual cell lines is regulated by the availability of a precursor, the expression level of β1,4-N-acetylgalactosaminyltransferase, α2,8-sialyltransferase activity and the compartmentation of the glycosylation machinery of a cell [80, 82]. Total ganglioside level has been shown to be a potential tool for evaluating the response to immunotherapy in melanoma patients [83, 84]. Furthermore, GM3 and GD3 shed by tumour cell into the microenvironment enhance tumour formation and are able to promote severe immune dysfunction [85–87]. At present, a number of gangliosides are considered to be attractive targets for cancer immunotherapy. GM3 is the precursor of the ganglioside family members that contain either N-glycolylneuraminic acid (Neu5Gc) or N-acetylneuraminic acid (Neu5Ac). The presence of Neu5Gc is a result of the expression of cytidine monophospho-N-acetylneuraminic acid hydrolase [88]. Although Neu5Gc-containing gangliosides are not self-antigens in humans [89], they have been described as tumour antigens in several human cancers including melanoma, lung and breast cancer [90–92]. The presence of Neu5GcGM3 on the cell membrane has been shown to promote cell proliferation and adhesion *in vitro* as well as tumour growth *in vivo* [93, 94]. Thus, Neu5GcGM3 are regarded as attractive targets for cancer immunotherapy [95]. Indeed, NeuGc5GM3-based vaccine composed of very small size proteoliposomes (VSSP) resulting from the hydrophobic conjunction of GM3 gangliosides with *Neisseria meningitides* membrane protein used in mice bearing early-stage B16-F10 melanoma tumours induced a complete anti-tumour protection in all mice [86, 93, 94]. Moreover, 1E10 monoclonal antibody, a murine anti-idiotypic antibody that mimics Neu5GcGM3, has been tested in several clinical trials for melanoma, breast and lung cancer as an anti-idiotypic cancer vaccine [96]. Also GD3, the most abundant ganglioside, has been used as an immunogen for trial vaccination against malignant melanoma [97]. Moreover, 9-O-acetylation of sialic acid containing gangliosides, especially 9-O-Ac-GD3 in human melanoma cells, provides a unique antigenic determinant, which is absent in normal human melanocytes [98]. Additionally, O-acetylated sialic acid residues reduce susceptibility of tumour cells to degradation and extend their lifetime *in vivo,* as well as may stimulate cellular growth and suppress cellular differentiation [99].

One of the important basic features of melanoma cells is the property to change their adhesive interactions with other cells (keratinocytes, fibroblasts, endothelial and immune cells) and extracellular matrix protein. This property is a key element in the acquisition of the potential to detach from their original site of tumour growth, invade surrounding tissues and, finally, metastasise. These interactions are mediated by cell adhesion molecules belonging to integrins, cadherins as well as immunoglobulin (Ig) superfamily. Changes in the expression and/or function of integrins, cadherins, CD44, Mel-CAM/MUC18 and intercellular adhesion molecule -1 have been documented in the progression of primary melanoma [100, 101]. It is also well documented in the literature that changes in cell adhesion molecules and growth factor receptors as a consequence of their oligosaccharide modification are associated with the function and biological behaviour of cancer cells. In the case of the cell surface receptors, the changed glycosylation pattern may affect their conformational stability, binding ability as well as their presence in the cell membrane. Details on changes in glycosylation patterns of cadherins and integrins that can modify the adhesive properties of melanoma cells are presented in two other chapters of this book.

The function of CD44, a widely distributed membrane glycoprotein belonging to the Ig superfamily, which abnormal expression on tumour cells enhances the ability to grow and metastasise *in vivo*, has been demonstrated to be partially influenced by O-linked oligosaccharides added to Ser/Thr-rich regions encoded by variable spliced CD44 exons [102]. In addition, all potential N-glycosylation sites in CD44 molecule have been proved to be necessary to maintain hyaluronic acid-recognition domain in the appropriate conformation [103]. Moreover, glycosylation of CD44 due to GnT-III enhanced B16-hm melanoma cell adhesion to hyaluronan, local tumour growth and metastatic growth in the spleen [104]. Other studies have shown that the presence of LAMP-1 with polylactosamine moieties on the cell surface of melanoma cells mediated organ-specific metastasis via lectin receptors on the lung vascular endothelium [105]. It has also been demonstrated that binding of a soluble ligand of SHPS-1 (i.e. CD47) to B16-F10 mouse melanoma cells was dependent on proper glycosylation of SHPS-1 molecule, another member of Ig superfamily, which plays an important role in integrin-mediated cytoskeleton reorganisation and migration, and that this defect renders melanoma cells resistant to CD47-induced inhibition of cell motility [106]. Interestingly, it has also been shown by deletion mutants that for P-glycoprotein function, which is a large and heavily glycosylated membrane protein conferring multi-drug resistance by pumping out a range of different drugs from the cell, N-glycosylation was necessary for its proper routing or stability but not for drug transport [107]. It is known that progression of melanoma correlates with the enhanced expression of glucose-regulated protein of 78 kDa (GRP78) and the increase in anti-GRP78 IgG serum titres in patients [108]. It has been shown that the glycosylation of anti-GRP-78 IgG changes as the disease progresses and the hyperglycosylated auto-antibodies stimulated cell proliferation via Akt signalling pathways [108].

It is well known that cancer metastases show organ selectivity and one of the important factors that determines the selectivity is the affinity of tumour cells towards the cells of an organ involved in metastasis. Most of the cell lines expressing β1,6-branched N-glycans have been shown to metastasise either to the liver or to the lung. β1,6-branched N-glycans are the preferred intermediate for the extension with polylactosamine chains (i.e. Galβ1,4GlcNAc β1,3- repeating units of 2 to more than 10 in length). Polylactosamine chains can be capped with various sequences, including Lewis antigens, sialic acids and fucose residues. It has been shown that lysosomal-associated membrane protein 1 (LAMP-1) present on the cell surface of high-metastatic murine B16-F10 cells was a carrier of a very high level of β1,6-branched N-glycans substituted with polylactosamine chains [105]. These structures were proved to be the key determinants in B16-F10 cells for preferred metastasising to the lungs, and organ-specific adhesion and metastasis was mediated via galectin-3 expressed in the highest amount on the lung vascular endothelium [105, 109, 110]. Complexes of galectin-3 with β1,6-branched N-glycans substituted with polylactosamine facilitated not only the initial arrest, but also took part in all the subsequent steps of extravasation and organ colonisation. Lung colonisation may also be realised by E-selectin-mediated interaction, but B16-F10 cells did not appear to use this molecule. B16-F10 cells transfected with cDNA encoding both α1,3- and α1,4-fucosyltransferases that catalyse reactions leading to the synthesis of sialyl-Lewis X and sialyl-Lewis A antigens, respectively, were not able to form metastasis in the liver in C57BL/6 mice, but formed numerous liver metastasis in E-selectin transgenic mice [111]. This means that sialyl-Lewis X (SAα2,3Galβ1,4(Fucα1,3)GlcNAcβ-) antigens on β1,6-branched N-glycans extended with polylactosamine chains did not serve as the ligand for lung colonisation in B16-F10 cells [105]. Human melanocytes did not express sialyl-Lewis X antigens and poorly expressed sialyl-Lewis A (SAα2,3Galβ1,3(Fucα1,4)GlcNAcβ-) antigens; however, these structures are overexpressed on cultured melanoma cells and melanoma tissue biopsies [112]. These findings indicated that sialyl-Lewis X and sialyl-Lewis A antigens are neoplastic differentiation antigens of human melanoma. Moreover, it has been proved that acquiring the expression level of sialyl-Lewis X antigens through the transfection of α1,3-fucosyltransferase III dramatically increased the metastatic capability of human melanoma McWo and mouse melanoma B16 cells [113, 114]. However, T antigen, another potential ligand for galectin-3, has not been involved in mouse lung-specific metastasis [109]. Nevertheless, α 2,3-linked sialic acids on the surface of B16-F10 cells have been demonstrated to play an important role in lung metastasis [115]. The use of soyasaponin I, an inhibitor that reduces the expression of α 2,3-linked sialic acids, not only enhanced cell adhesion to extracellular matrix proteins, reduced cell migration, but also reduced the ability of melanoma cells for lung colonisation in mice. The positive correlation between the level of α1,6-fucosylated biantennary N-glycans on B16 murine cells and cellular potential to metastasise to the lung has been also demonstrated [116]. It has also been shown that cells expressing multi-antennary N-oligosaccharides un-substituted with polylactosamine chains home in the liver which expresses galectin-1 [117].

Recent advances in the discovery of microRNA (miRNA) role in cutaneous melanoma pathogenesis have revealed that miRNA can affect the cell surface proteins by interfering with their post-translational modifications. It has been found that overexpression of *miR-30b* and *miR-30d* in primary and metastatic tissues induced changes in glycosylation profiles of the membrane-bound proteins [118]. Moreover, *miR-30b* and *miR-30d* up-regulation was correlated with the stage, metastatic potential, shorter time to recurrence and reduced overall survival. *GALNT7* was found to be the specific gene target that mediated these pro-metastatic effects. GALNT7 belongs to GalNAc transferases, which initiate mucin-type O-linked glycosylation in the Golgi apparatus [119]. Another consequence of *miR-30b* and *miR-30d* overexpression was the reduction of CD3+ T cells recruitment and accumulation of regulatory T cells at the metastatic site *in vivo*, which could be partially mediated by increased secretion of IL-10. Thus, targeting *miR-30b/30d* in melanoma cells could counteract both with its pro-metastatic and immunosuppressive effects by de-repressing GALNT7 endogenous level.

To date, one monoclonal antibody TM10 produced from mice vaccinated with FasL-expressing B16-F10 mouse melanoma cells was able to recognise a range of human tumour cell lines, including melanoma [120]. Despite the fact that over 50% of cancers express tumour-associated carbohydrate antigens, such as gangliosides, Lewis antigens and Thomsen-Friedenreich antigen, none of them was the antigenic target of TM10. However, another monoclonal antibody HMB45 that recognises melanoma-specific target, i.e. Pmel17/gp100, reacts with its sialylated RPT domain [121].

4. Glycation and melanoma

The risk of melanoma is significantly associated with high fasting glucose, which is entirely independent on age, body mass index and smoking [122]. A non-enzymatic reaction (glycation) between ketones or aldehydes and amino groups of proteins contributes to the ageing of proteins and leads to the formation and accumulation of irreversible cross-linked protein derivatives termed advanced glycation end products (AGE). AGE have been proved to stimulate growth and migration of malignant melanoma *in vitro* and *in vivo* through the interaction with the receptor for advanced glycation end products (RAGE) [123–126]. RAGE is known to stimulate multiple signalling pathways crucial for cell migration, such as p38 mitogen-activated protein kinase, Ras-extracellular signal-regulated kinase 1/2, stress-activated protein kinase/c-Jun-NH2-terminal kinase and Cdc42/Rac pathways. Recently, RAGE expressed on mouse melanoma B16 cells has been identified as a crucial factor for pulmonary metastases of these tumour cells [127]. Interestingly, RAGE has also been identified as a potential anti-metastatic drug target [128].

RAGE has been shown to interact with S100B [129], which is a serological biomarker widely used in clinical practice to determine the prognosis for patients with distal melanoma metastases, despite the fact that it fails to detect melanoma progression in up to 20% of patients [130–133]. Recently, it has been demonstrated that among stage III–IV melanoma patients, decreased serum levels of soluble forms of RAGE (sRAGE and esRAGE) correlated with poor overall survival [134]. Interestingly, it has also been proved that overexpression of RAGE in WM115 human primary melanoma cells was associated with mesenchymal-like morphology of the cell, a switch to a metastatic phenotype as well as up-regulation of S100B [126]. As the elevated level of S100B is known to down-regulate p53 suppressor protein, small-molecule inhibitors targeting S100B-p53 interaction are currently under intense investigations as new therapeutic strategies for malignant melanoma [135, 136]. It has also been shown that the expression of S100P, which is another member of the S100 family, was significantly higher in malignant melanoma than in primary melanoma [137]. Abnormal level of S100P can contribute to tumour growth, invasion and metastasis [138]. Other functional ligands for RAGE include chondroitin sulphate containing E disaccharide units (GlcNAβ1-3GalNAc(4,6-O-disulfate)β1-) and heparin sulphate [127].

5. Conclusions

Alterations in glycans on proteins and lipids have long been associated with malignant transformation. The observed modifications are either a direct consequence of the oncogenic process or an indirect effect of changes occurring in the tissue environment and inflammation. Analytical efforts in melanoma glycomics contribute to understanding the role of cellular and molecular properties of cells that influence the dissemination of tumour cells, which might be essential for understanding the pathogenesis of tumour development and metastasis. These studies also offer considerable possibilities for screening, selection and identification of differentially expressed glycoconjugates, in order to develop non-invasive, sensitive and discriminative *in vitro* diagnostics tests. Unfortunately, the vast majority of studies have been performed on melanoma cell lines and mouse model systems due to the insufficient number of samples obtained from melanoma patients. Therefore, there is still limited evidence on whether the observations made in these models are consistent with the role of glycosylation in tumour tissues. Further studies based on human tissues are needed to establish functional impact of glycosylation changes on human melanoma as well as detection and discovery of glycan motifs in melanoma samples similarly to advances achieved in lung, liver, colorectal, brain, prostate, breast and ovarian cancer researches.

Acknowledgements

The writing of this manuscript was supported in part by grants from the Institute of Zoology, Jagiellonian University in Krakow (K/ZDS/005403) and from the National Science Centre, Poland (2013/11/B/NZ4/04315).

Author details

Małgorzata Przybyło*, Marcelina E. Janik and Dorota Hoja-Łukowicz

*Address all correspondence to: malgorzata.przybylo@uj.edu.pl

Department of Glycoconjugate Biochemistry, Institute of Zoology, Jagiellonian University, Kraków, Poland

References

[1] Garbe C, Leiter U: Melanoma epidemiology and trends. Clin Dermatol. 2009;27:3–9. DOI: 10.1016/j.clindermatol.2008.09.001

[2] Erdmann F, Lortet-Tieulent J, Schüz J, Zeeb H, Greinert R, Breitbart EW, Bray F: International trends in the incidence of malignant melanoma 1953-2008 – are recent generations at higher of lower risk? Int J Cancer. 2013;132:385–400. DOI: 10.1002/ijc.27616

[3] Dummer R, Hauschild A, Jost L: Cutaneous malignant melanoma: ESMO clinical recommendations for diagnosia, treatment and follo-up. Anna Oncol. 2008;19:86–88. DOI: 10.1093/annonc/mdn100

[4] Garbe C, Peris K, Hauschild A, Saiag P, Middeleton M, Spaza A, Grob JJ, Malvehy J, Newton-Bishop J, Stratigos A, Pehamberger H, Eggermont A: Diagnosis and treatment of melanoma: European consensus-based interdisciplinary guideline. Eur J Cancer. 2010;46:270–283. DOI: 10.1016/j.ejca.2009.10.032

[5] Ohtsubo K, Marth JD: Glycosylation in cellular mechanisms of health and disease. Cell. 2006;126:855–867

[6] Varki ACR, Cummings R, Esko JD, Freeze HH, Stanley P, Bertozzi CR, Hart GW, Etzler ME, editors. Essentials of Glycobiology. 2nd edition. Cold Spring Harbor (NY): Cold Spring Harbor Laboratory Press; 2009.

[7] Jankowic M: Glycans as biomarkers: status and perspectives. J Med Biochem. 2011;30:213–223. DOI: 10.2478/v10011-011-0023-5

[8] Moremen KW, Tiemeyer M, Nairn AV: Vertebrate protein glycosylation: diversity, synthesis and function. Nat Rev Mol Cell Biol. 2012;13:448–462. DOI: 10.1038/nrm3383

[9] Adamczyk B, Tharmalingam T, Rudd PM: Glycans as cancer biomarkers. Biochem Biophys Acta. 2012;1820:1347–1353. DOI: 10.1016/j.bbagen.2011.12.001

[10] Hennet T: Disease of glycosylation beyond classical congenital disorders of glycosylation. Biochim Biophys Acta. 2012;1820:1306–1317. DOI: 10.1016/j.bbagen.2012.02.001

[11] Freire-de-Lima L: Sweet and sour: the impact of differentia glycosylation in cancer cell understanding epithelial-mesenchymal transition. Front Oncol. 2014;5:59. DOI: 10.3389/fonc.2014.00059

[12] Taniguchi N, Kizuka Y: Glycans and cancer: role of N-glycans in cancer biomarker, progression and metastasis, and therapeutics. Adv Cancer Res. 2015;126:11–52. DOI: 10.1016/bs.acr.2014.11.001

[13] Spiro R: Protein glycosylation: nature, distribution, enzymatic formation, and disease implication of glycopeptide bonds. Glycobiology. 2002;12:43–56.

[14] Knezevic A, Gornik O, Polasek O, Pucic M, Redzic I, Novokmet M, Rudd PM, Wright AF, Campbell H, Rudan I, Lauc G: Effect of aging, body mass index, plasma lipid profiles, and smoking on human plasma N-glycans. Glycobiology. 2010;20:959–969. DOI: 10.1093/glycob/cwq051

[15] Strowell SR, Ju T, Cummings RD: Protein glycosylation in cancer. Annu Rev Pathol. 2015;10:473–510. DOI: 10.1146/annurev-pathol-012414-040438

[16] Vojta A, Samaržija I, Bočkor L, Zoldoš V: Glyco-gene change expression in cancer through aberrant methylation. Biochim Biophys Acta. 2016:1860:1776–1785. DOI: 10.1016/j.bbagen.2016.01.002

[17] Dennis JW, Granovsky M, Warren CE: Glycoprotein glycosylation and cancer progression. Biochim Biophys Acta. 1999;1473:21–34.

[18] Fuster MM, Esko JD: The sweet and sour of cancer: glycans as novel therapeutic targets. Nat Rev Cancer. 2005;5:526–542.

[19] Wandall H, Tarp MA: Therapeutic cancer vaccines: clinical trials and applications. In: Guo Z, Boons GJ, editors. Carbohydrate-based Vaccines and Immunotherapies. Hoboken, New Jersey: Wiley & Sons Inc; 2009. pp. 333–366. DOI: 10.1002/9780470473283.ch10

[20] Markidakis M, Vlahou A: Secretome proteomics for discovery of cancer biomarkers. J Proteom. 2010;73:2291–2305. DOI: 10.1016/j.jprot.2010.07.001

[21] Shukla HD, Vaitiekunas P, Cotter RJ: Advances in membrane proteomics and cancer biomarker discovery: Currant status and future prespective. Proteomics. 2012;12:3085–3104. DOI: 10.1002.pmic.201100519

[22] Christiansen MN, Chik JJ, Lee L, Anugraham M, Abrahams JL, Packer NH: Cell surface glycosylation in cancer. Proteomics. 2014;14:525–546. DOI: 10.1002/pmic.201300387

[23] De la Luz-Hernandez K, Rabas Y, Monlesinos R, Fuentes D, Santo-Tomás JF, Morales O, Aquilar Y, Pacheco B, Castillo A: Cancer vaccine characterisation: From bench to clinic. Vaccine 2014;32:2851–2858. DOI: 10.1016/j.vaccine.2014.02.017

[24] Padler-Karavani V: Aiming at the sweet side of cancer: aberrant glycosylation as possible target for personalized-medicine. Cancer Lett. 2014;352:102–112. DOI: 10.1016/j.canlet.2013.10.005

[25] Rho JH, Mead JR, Wright WS, Brenner DE, Stave JW, Gildersleeve JC, Lampe PD: Discovery of sialyl Lewis A and Lewis X modified protein cancer biomarkers using high density antibody arrays. J Proteomics. 2014;96:291–299. DOI: 10.1016/j.jprot.2013.10.030

[26] Zhang X, Wang Y, Qian Y, Wu X, Zhang Z, Liu X, Zhao R, Zhou L, Ruan Y, Xu J, Liu H, Ren S, Xu C, Gu J: Discovery of specific metastasis-related N-glycan alterations in epithelial ovarian cancer based on quantitative glycomics. PLoS One. 2014;9:e87978. DOI: 10.1371/journal.pone.0087978

[27] Packer NH, von der Lieth CW, Aoki-Kinoshita KF, Lebrilla CB, Paulson JC, Raman R, Rudd P, Sasisekharan R, Taniguchi N, York WS: Frontiers in glycomics: bioinformatics and biomarker in disease. An NIH white paper prepared from discussions by the focus

group at a workshop on the NIH campus, Bethesda, MD (September 11–13, 2006). Proteomics. 2008;8:8–20.

[28] Gu J, Taniguchi N: Potential of N-glycan in cell adhesion and migration either a positive or negative regulator. Cell Adh Migr. 2008;2:243–245.

[29] Kufe DW: Mucins in cancer: function, prognosis and therapy. Nat Rev. 2009; 9:631–664. DOI: 10.1038/nrc2761

[30] Gu J, Isaji T, Xu Q, Kariya Y, Gu W, Fukuda T, Du Y: Potential roles of N-glycosylation in cell adhesion. Glycoconj J. 2012;29:599–607. DOI: 10.1007/s10719-012-9386

[31] Pinho SS, Oliveira P, Cabral J, Carvalho S, Huntsman D, Gärtner F, Seruca R, Reis CA, Oliveira C: Loss and recovery of Mgat3 and GnT-III mediated E-cadherin N-glycosylation is a mechanism involved in epithelial-mesenchymal-epithelial transition. PLoS One. 2012;7:e33191. DOI: 10.1371/journal.pone.0033191

[32] Li N, Xu H, Fan K, Liu X, Qi J, Zhao C, Yin P, Wang L, Li Z, Zha X: Altered β1,6-GlcNAC branched N-glycans impair TGF-β-mediated epithelial-to-mesenchymal transition through Smad signalling pathway in human lung cancer. J Cell Mol Med. 2014;18:1975–1991. DOI: 10.1111/jcmm.12331

[33] Radhakrishnan P, Dabelsteen S, Madsen FB, Francavilla C, Kopp KL, Steentoft C, Vahhrushev SY, Olsen JV, Hansen L, Bennet EP, Woetmann A, Yin G, Chen L, Song H, Bak M, Hlady RA, Peters SL, Opavsky R, Thode C, Qvortrup K, Schjoldager KT, Clausen H, Hollingsworth MA, Wandall HH: Immature truncated O-glycophenotype of cancer directly induces oncogenic features. Proc Natl Acad Sci U S A. 2014;111:E4066-75. DOI: 10.1073/pnas.1406619111

[34] Tan Z, Lu W, Li X, Yang G, Guo J, Yu H, Li Z, Guan F: Alteed N-glycan expression profile in epithelial-to-mesenchymaltransition of NMuMG cells revealed by an integrated strategy using mass spectrometry and glycogene and lectin microarray analysis. J Proteome Res. 2014;13:2783–2795. DOI: 10.1021/pr401185z

[35] Herlyn M, Fukunaga-Kalabis M: What is a good model for melanoma? J Invest Dermatol. 2010;130:911–912. DOI: 10.1038/jid.2009.441

[36] Passaniti A, Hart GW: Cell surface sialylation and tumor metastasis. Metastatic potential of B16 melanoma variants correlates with their relative number of specific penultimate oligosaccharide structures. J Biol Chem. 1988;263:7591–7603.

[37] Finne J, Tao TW, Burger MM: Carbohydrate changes in glycoproteins of a poorly metastasizing wheat germ agglutinin-resistant melanoma clone. Cancer Res. 1980;40:25802587.

[38] Burger MM, Tao TW, Finne J, Prieels JP: The influence of membrane mutations on metastasis. Biosci Rep. 1982;2:597–599.

[39] Gorelik E, Duty L, Anakari F, Galili U: Alterations of cell surface carbohydrates and inhibition of metastatic property of murine melanomas by alpha 1,3 galactosyltransferasegene expression. Melanoma Res. 1995;55:4168–4173.

[40] Tulsiani DRP, Harris TM, Touster O: Swainsonine inhibits the biosynthesis of complex glycoproteins by inhibition of Golgi α-mannosidase II. J Biol Chem. 1982;257:7936–7939.

[41] Humphries MJ, Matsumoto K, White SL, Olden K: Oligosaccharide modification by swainsonine treatment inhibits pulmonary colonization by B16F10 murine melanoma cells. Proc Natl Acad Sci U S A. 1986;S3:1752–2756.

[42] Dennis JW, Koch K, Yousefi S, VanderElst: Growth inhibition of human melanoma tumor xenografts in athymic nude mice by swainsonine. Cancer Res. 1990;50:1867–1872.

[43] Goss PE, Reid CL, Bailey D, Dennis JW: Phase IB clinical trial of the oligosaccharide processing inhibitor swainsonine in patients with advanced malignancies. Clin Cancer Res. 1997;3:1077–1086.

[44] Yoshimura M, Nishikawa A, Ihara Y, Taniguchi S, Taniguchi N: Suppression of lung metastasis of B16 mouse melanoma by N-acetylglucosaminyltransferase III gene transfection. Proc Natl Acad Sci USA. 1995;92:8754–8758.

[45] Yoshimura M, Ihera Y, Matsuzawa Y, Taniguchi N: Abberant glycosylation of E-cadherin enhances cell-cell binging to suppress metastasis. J Biol Chem. 1996;271:3811–3815.

[46] Dricu A, Carlberg M, Wang M, Larsson O: Inhibition of N-linked glycosylation using tunicamycin causes cell death in malignant cells: role of down regulation of the insulin-like growth factor 1 receptor in induction of apoptosis. Cancer Res. 1997;57:543–548.

[47] Dricu A, Wang M, Hjertman M, Malec M, Blegen H, Wejde J, Carlberg M, Larsson O: Mevalonate-regulated mechanizms in cell growth control: role of dolichyl phosphate in expression of the insulin-like growth factor-1 receptor (IGF-IR) in comparison to Ras prenylation and expression of c-myc. Glycobiology. 1997:7:625–633.

[48] Przybyło M, Martuszewska D, Pocheć E, Hoja-Łukowicz D, Lityńska A: Identification of proteins bearing β1-6 branched N-glycans In human melanoma cell lines from different progression stages by tandem mass spectrometry analysis. Biochim Biophys Acta. 2007;1770:1427–1435.

[49] Taniguchi N, Korekane H: Branched N-glycans and their implications for cell adhesion, signaling and clinical application for cancer biomarkers and in therapeutics. BMB Rep. 2011;44:772–781.

[50] Gorelik E, Galili U, Raz A: On the role of cell surface carbohydrates and their binding proteins (lectins) in tumor metastasis. Cancer Metastasis Rev. 2001;20:245–277.

[51] Chakraborty AK, Pawelek J, Ikeda Y, Miyoshi E, Kolesnimova N, Funasaka Y, Ichihashi M, Taniguchi N: Fusion hybrids with macrophage and melanoma cells up-regulate N-acetylglucosaminyltransferase V, β1-6 branching, and metastasis. Cell Growth Differ. 2001;12:623–630.

[52] Pawelek JM: Viewing malignant melanoma cells as macrophage tumor hybrids. Cell Adh Migr. 2007;1:2–6.

[53] Pawelek JM, Chakraborty AK: The cancer cell-leucocyte fusion theory of metastasis. Adv Cancer Res. 2008;101:397–444. DOI: 10.1016/S0065-230X(08)00410-7

[54] Lazova R, Pawelek JM: Why melanomas get so dark? Exp Dermatol. 2009;18:934–938. DOI: 10.1111/j.1600-0625.2009.00933.x

[55] Lazova R, Klump V, Pawelek J: Autophagy in cutaneous malignant melanoma. J Cutan Pathol. 2010;37:256–268. DOI: 10.1111/j.1600-0560.2009.01359.x

[56] Granovsky M, Fata J, Pawling J, Muller WJ, Khokha R, Dennis JW: Supression of tumor growth and metastasis in Mgat5-deficient mice. Nature. 2000;6:306–312.

[57] Lityńska A, Przybyło M, Pocheć E, Hoja-Łukowicz D, Ciołczyk D, Laidler P, Gil D: Comparison of the lectin-binding pattern in different human melanoma cell lines. Melanoma Res. 2001;11:201–212.

[58] Mendoza I, Olaso E, Anasagasti MJ, Fuentes AM, Vidal-Vanaclocha F: Mannose receptor-mediated endothelial activation contributes to B16 melanoma cell adhesion and metastasis in liver. J Cell Physiol. 1998;174:322–330.

[59] Laidler P, Lityńska A, Hoja-Łukowicz D, Łabędź M, Przybyło M, Ciołczyk-Wierzbicka D, Pocheć E, Trębacz E, Kremser E: Characterization of glycosylation and adherent properties of melanoma cells. Cancer Immunol Immuther. 2006;55:112–118. DOI: 10.1007/s00262-005-0019-4

[60] Pocheć E, Janik M, Hoja-Łukowicz D, Link-Lenczowski P, Przybyło M, Lityńska A: Expression of integrins α3β1 and α5β1 and GlcNAc β 1,6 glycan branching influences metastatic melanoma cell migration on fibronectin. Eur J Cell Biol. 2013;92:355–362. DOI: 10.1016/j.ejcb.2013.10.007

[61] Handerson T, Berger A, Harigopol M, Rimm D, Nishigori C, Ueda M, Miyoshi E, Taniguchi N, Pawelek J: Melanophages reside in hypermelanotic, aberrantly glycosylated tumor areas and predict improved outcome in primary cutaneous malignant melanoma. J Clin Pathol. 2007;34:679–686. DOI: 10.1111/j.1600-0560.2006.00681

[62] Litynska A, Przybylo M, Pochec E, Kremser E, Hoja-Lukowicz D, Sulowska U: Does glycosylation of melanoma cells influence their interaction with fibronectin? Biochimie. 2006;88:527–534.

[63] Przybyło M, Pocheć E, Link-Lenczowski P, Lityńska A: β1-6 branching of cell surface glycoproteins may contribute to uveal melanoma progression by up-regulating cell motility. Mol Vis. 2008;14:625–636.

[64] Krähling H, Mally S, Eble JA, Noël J, Schwab A, Stock C: The glycocalyx maintains a cell surface pH nanoenvironment crucial for integrin-mediated migration of human melanoma cells. Pflugers Arch. 2009;458:1069–1083. DOI: 10.1007/s00424-009-0694-7

[65] Ochwat D, Hoja-Łukowicz D, Lityńska A: N-glycoproteins bearing β1-6 branched oligosaccharides from the A375 human melanoma cell line analysed by tandem mass spectrometry. Melanoma Res. 2004;14:479–485.

[66] Pocheć E, Lityńska A, Amoresano A, Casbarra A: Glycosylation profile of integrin α3β1 integrin changes with melanoma progression. Biochim Biophys Acta. 2003;1644:113–123.

[67] Ciołczyk-Wierzbicka D, Amoresano A, Casbarr A, Hoja-Łukowicz D, Lityńska A, Laidler P: The structure of the oligosaccharides of N-cadherin from human melanoma cell lines. Glycoconjugate J. 2004;20:483–492.

[68] Kremser ME, Przybyło M, Hoja-Łukowicz D, Pocheć E, Amoresano A, Carpentieri A, Bubka M, Lityńska A: Characterisation of α3β1 and αvβ3 integrin N-oligosaccharides in metastatic melanoma WM9 and WM239 cell lines. Biochim Biophys Acta. 2008;1780:1421–1431. DOI: 10.1016/j.bbagen.2008.07.011

[69] Janik ME, Przybyło M, Pocheć E, Pokrywka M, Lityńska A: Effect of α3β1 and αvβ3 integrin glycosylation on interaction of melanoma cells with vitronectin. Acta Biochim Pol. 2010;57:55–61.

[70] Hoja-Łukowicz D, Link-Lenczowski P, Carpentieri A, Amoresano A, Pocheć E, Artemenko K, Bergquist J, Lityńska A: L1CAM from human melanoma carries a novel type of N-glycan with Galβ1-4Galβ1- motif. Involvement of N-linked glycans in migratory and invasive behaviour of melanoma cells. Glycoconj J. 2013;30:205–225. DOI: 10.1007/s10719-012-9374-5

[71] Janik ME, Lityńska A, Przybyło M: Studies on primary uveal and cutaneous melanoma cell interaction with vitronectin. Cell Biol Int. 2014;38:942–952. DOI: 10.1002/cbin.10280

[72] Taniguchi N, Miyoshi E, Jianguo G, Honke K, Matsumoto A: Decoding sugar function by identifying target glycoproteins. Curr Opin Struct Biol. 2006;16:561–566.

[73] Thies A, Moll I, Berger J, Schumacher U: Lectin binding to cutaneous malignant melanoma: HPA is associated with metastasis formation. Br J Cancer. 2001;84:819–823.

[74] Singhal A, Fohn M, Hakomori S: Induction of α-N-acetylgalactosamine-O-serine/threonine (Tn) antigen-mediated cellular response for active immunotherapy in mice. Cancer Res. 1991;51:1406–1411.

[75] Hoja-Łukowicz D, Przybyło P, Pocheć E, Drabik A, Silberring J, Kremser M, Schadendorf D, Laidler P, Lityńska A: The new face of nucleolin in human melanoma. Cancer Immunol Immunother. 2009;58:1471–1480. DOI: 10.1007/s00262-009-0705-8

[76] Ostankovitch M, Altrich-VanLith M, Robila V, Engelhard VH: N-glycosylation enhances presentation of a MHC class I-restricted epitope from tyrosinase. J Immunol. 2009;182:4830–4835. DOI: 10.4049/jimmunol.0802902

[77] Kittlesen DJ, Thompson LW, Gulden PH, Skipper JC, Colella TA, Shabanowitz JA, Hunt DF, Engelhard VH, Slingluff Jr CL: Human melanoma patients recognize an HLA-A1-restricted CTL epitope from tyrosinase containing two cysteine residues: implications for tumor vaccine development. J Immunol. 1998; 160:2099–2106.

[78] Passaniti A, Hart GW: Metastasis-associated murine melanoma cell surface galactosyltransferase: characterisation of enzyme activity and identification of major surface substrates. Cancer Res. 1990;50:7261–7271.

[79] Ruan S, Lioyd KO: Glycosylation pathways in the biosynthesis of gangliosides in melanoma and neuroblastoma cells: relative glycosyltransferase levels determine ganglioside patterns. Cancer Res. 1992;52:5725–5731.

[80] Yamashiro S, Ruan S, Furukawa K, Tai T, Lloyd KO, Shiku H, Furukawa K: Genetic and enzymatic basis for the differential expression of GM2 and GD2 gangliosides in human cancer cell lines. Cancer Res. 1993;53:5395–5400.

[81] Morton DL, Ravindranath MH, Irie RF: Tumor gangliosides as targets for active specific immunotherapy of melanoma in men. Prog Brain Res. 1994;101:251–275.

[82] Yamashiro S, Haraguchi M, Furukawa K, Takamiya K, Yamamoto A, Nagata Y, Lloyd KO, Shiku H, Furukawa K: Substrate specificity of β1,4 N-acetylgalactosaminyltransferase in vitro and in cDNA-transfected cells. GM2/GD2 synthase efficiently generates asialo-GM2 in certain cells. J Biol Chem. 1995;270:6149–6155.

[83] Ravindranath MH, Hsueh EC, Verma M, Ye W, Morton DL: Serum total ganglioside level correlates with clinical course in melanoma patients after immunotherapy with therapeutic cancer vaccine. J Immunother. 2003;26:277–285.

[84] Kavanagh D, Hill AD, Djikstra B, Kennelly R, McDermott EM, O'Higgins NJ: Adjuvant therapies in the treatment of stage II and III malignant melanoma. Surgeon. 2005;3:245–256.

[85] Ladisch S, Kitada S, Hays EF: Gangliosides shed by tumor cells enhance tumor formation in mice. J Clin Invest. 1987;79:1879–1882.

[86] Carr A, Mazorra Z, Alonso DF, Mesa C, Valiente O, Gomez DE, Perez R, Fernandez LE: A purified GM3 ganglioside conjugated vaccine induces specific, adjuvant-dependent and non-transient antitumour activity against B16 mouse melanoma in vitro and in vivo. Melanoma Res. 2001;11:219–227.

[87] Bennaceur K, Popa I, Portoukalian J, Berthier-Vergnes O, Péguet-Navarro J: Melanoma-derived gangliosides impair migratory and antigen-presenting function of human epidermal Langerhans cells and induce their apoptosis. Int Immunol. 2006;18:879–886.

[88] Shaw L, Schauer R: The biosynthesis of N-glycoloylneuraminic acid occurs by hydroxylation of the CMP-glycoside of N-acetylneuraminic acid. Biol Chem Hoppe Seyler. 1988;369:477–486.

[89] Irie A, Koyama S, Kozutsumi Y, Kawasaki T, Suzuki A: The molecular basis for the absence of N-glycolylneuraminic acid in humans. J Biol Chem. 1998; 273:15866–15871.

[90] Malykh YN, Schauer R, Shaw L: N-Glycolylneuraminic acid in human tumours. Biochimie. 2001;83:623–634.

[91] Carr A, Mullet A, Mazorra Z, Vazquez AM, Alfonso M, Mesa C, Rengifo E, Perez R, Fernandez LE: A mouse IgG1 monoclonal antibody specific for N-glycolyl GM3 ganglioside recognized breast and melanoma tumors. Hybridoma. 2000;19:241–247.

[92] Fernandez A, Mesa C, Marigo I, Dolcetti L, Clavell M, Oliver L, Fernandez LE, Bronte V: Inhibition of tumor-induced myeloid-derived suppressor cell function by nanoparticulated adjuvant. J Immunol. 2011;186:264–274. DOI: 10.4049/jimmunol.1001465

[93] Gabri MR, Mazorra Z, Ripoll GV, Mesa C, Fernandez LE, Gomez DE, Alonso DF: Complete antitumor protection by perioperative immunization with GM3/VSSP vaccine in a preclinical mouse melanoma model. Clin Cancer Res. 2006;12:7092–7098.

[94] Segatori VI, Otero LL, Fernandez LE, Gomez DE, Alonso DF, Gabri MR: Antitumor protection by NGcGM3/VSSP vaccine against transfected B16 mouse melanoma cell overexpression N-glycolylated gangliosides. In Vivo. 2012;26:609–617.

[95] de Leon J, Fernandez A, Mesa C, Clavel M, Fernandez LE: Role of tumour associated N-glycolylated variant of GM3 ganglioside in cancer progression: effect over CD4 expression on T cells. Cancer Immunol Immunother. 2006;55:443–450.

[96] Machado YJ, Rabasa Y, Montesinos R, Cremata J, Besada V, Fuentes D, Castillo A, de la Luz KR, Vázquez AM, Himly M: Physicochemical and biological characterization of 1E10 anti-idiotype vaccine. BMC Biotechnol. 2011;11:12. DOI: 10.1186/1472-6750-11-112

[97] Ragupathi G, Meyers M, Adluri S, Howard L, Musselli C, Livingston PO: Induction of antibodies against GD3 ganglioside in melanoma patients by vaccination with GD3-lactone-KLH conjugate plus immunological adjuvant QS-21. Int J Cancer. 2000;85:659–666.

[98] Cheresh DA, Reisfeld RA, Varki AP: O-acetylation of disialoganglioside GD3 by human melanoma cells creates a unique antigenic determinant. Science. 1984;225:844–846.

[99] Kohla G, Stockfleth E, Schauer R: Gangliosides with O-acetylated sialic acids in tumors of neuroectodermal origin. Neurochem Res. 2002;27:583–592.

[100] Bogenrieder T, Herlyn M: Cell-surface proteolysis, growth factor activation and intracellular communication in the progression of melanoma. Crit Rev Oncol Hematol. 2002;44:1–15.

[101] Li G, Satayamoorthy K, Herlyn M: Dynamics of cell interactions and communication during melanoma development. Crit Rev Oral Biol Mol. 2002;13:62–70. DOI: 10.1111/j.1600-0560.2009.01359.x

[102] Bennet KL, Modrell B, Greenfield B, Bartolazzi A, Stamenkovic I, Peach R, Jackson DG, Spring F, Aruffo A: Regulation of CD44 binding to hyaluronan by glycosylation of variable spliced exons. J Cell Biol. 1995;131:1623–1633.

[103] Bartolazzi A, Nocks A, Aruffo A, Spring F, Stamenkovic I: Glycosylation of CD44 is implicated in CD44-mediated cell adhesion to hyaluronan. J Cell Biol. 1996;132:1199–1208.

[104] Sheng Y, Yoshimura M, Inouke S, Oritani K, Nishiura T, Yoshida H, Ogawa M, Okajima Y, Matsuzawa Y, Taniguchi N: Remodeling of glycoconjugates on CD44 enhances cell adhesion to hyaluronate, tumor growth and metastasis in B16 melanoma cees expressing β1,4-N-acetylglycosaminyltransferase III. Int J Cancer. 1997;73:850–858.

[105] Krishnan V, Bane SM, Kawle PD, Naresh KN, Kalraiya RD: Altered melanoma cell surface glycosylation mediates organ specific adhesion and metastasis via lectin receptors on the lung vascular endothelium. Clin Exp Metastasis. 2005;22:11–24.

[106] Ogura T, Noguchi T, Murai-Takebe R, Hosooka T, Honma N, Kasuga M: Resistance of B16 melanoma cells to CD47-induced negative regulation of motility as a result of aberrant N-glycosylation of SHPS-1. J Biol Chem. 2004;279:13711–13720.

[107] Schinkel AH, Kemp S, Dolle M, Rudenko G, Wagenaar E: N-glycosylation and deletion mutants of the human MDR1 P-glycoprotein. J Biol Chem. 1993;268:7474–7481

[108] Selim MA, Burchette JL, Bowers EV, de Ridder GG, Mo L, Pizzo SV, Gonzalez-Gronow M: Changes in oligosaccharide chains of autoantibodies of GRP78 expressed during progression of malignant melanoma stimulate melanoma cell growth and survival. Melanoma Res. 2011;21:323–334. DOI: 10.1097/CMR.0b013e3283471042

[109] Srinivasan N, Bane SM, Ahire SD, Ingle AD, Kalraiya RD: Poly-N-acetyllactosamine substitution on N- and nor O-oligosaccharides or Thomsen-Friedenreich antigen facilitate lung specific metastasis of melanoma cells via galectin-3. Glycocon J. 2009;26:445–456. DOI: 10.1007/s10719-008-9194-9

[110] More SK, Srinivasan N, Budnar S, Bane SM, Upadhya A, Thorat RA, Ingle AD, Chiplunkar SV, Kalraiya RD: N-glycans and metastasis in galectin-3 transgenic mice. Biochem Biophys Res Commun. 2015;460:302–307. DOI: 10.1016/j.bbrc.2015.03.030

[111] Biancone L, Araki M, Araki K, Vassalli P, Stamenkovic I: Redirection of tumor metastasis by expressing E-selectin in vivo. J Exp Med. 1996;183:581–587.

[112] Ravindranath MH, Amiri AA, Bauer PM, Kelley MC, Essner R, Morton DL: Endothelial-selectin ligands sialyl Lewis x and sialyl Lewis a are differentiation antigens immunogenic in human melanoma. Cancer. 1997;79:1686–1697.

[113] Ohyama C, Tsuboi S, Fukuda M: Dual roles of sialyl Lewis X oligosaccharides in tumor metastasis and rejection by natural killer cells. EMBO J. 1999;18:1516–1525.

[114] Ohyama C, Kanto S, Kato K, Nakano O, Arai Y, Kato T, Chen S, Fukuda MN, Fukuda M: Natural killer cells attack tumor cells expressing high levels of sialyl Lewis x oligosaccharides. PNAS. 2002;99:13789–13794.

[115] Chang WW, Yu CY, Lin TW, Wang PH, Tsai YC: Soyasaponin I decreases the expression α2,3-linked sialic acids on the cell surface and supresses the metastatic potential of B16F10 melanoma cells. Biochim Biophys Res Commun. 2006;341:614–619.

[116] Sakuma K, Fujimoto I, Hitoshi S, Tanaka F, Ikeda T, Tanabe K, Toyokuni S, Wada H, Mio T, Mishima M, Ikenaka K: An N-glycan structure correlates with pulmonary metastatic ability of cancer cells. Biochim Biophys Res Commun. 2006;340:829–835.

[117] Reddy BV, Kalraiya RD: Sialylated beta1,6 branched N-oligosaccharides modulate adhesion, chemotaxis and motility of melanoma cells: Effect on invasion and spontaneous metastasis properties. Biochim Biophys Acta 2006;1760:1393–1402.

[118] Gaziel-Sovran A, Segura MF, Di Micco R, Collins MK, Hanniford D, Vega-Saenz de Miera E, Rakus JF, Dankert JF, Shang S, Kerbel RS, Bhardwaj N, Shao Y, Darvishian F, Zavadil J, Erlebacher A, Mahal LK, Osman I, Hernando E. miR-30b/30d regulation of GalNAc transferase enhances invasion and immunosuppression during metastasis. Cancer Cell. 2011;20:104–118. DOI: 10.1016/j.ccr.2011.05.027

[119] Ten Hagen KG, Fritz TA, Tabak LA: All in the family: the UDP-GalNAc:polypeptide N-acetylgalactosaminyltransferases. Glycobiology. 2003;13:1R–16R

[120] Nowsom-Davis TE, Wang D, Stein L, Chen PFT, Wang LX, Simon AK, Screaton GR: Enhanced immune recognition of cryptic glycan markers in human tumors. Cancer Res. 2009;69:2018–2025. DOI: 10.1158/0008-5472.CAN-08-3589

[121] Hoashi T, Tamaki K, Hearing VJ: The secreted form of a melanocyte membrane-bound glycoprotein (Pmel17/gp100) is released by ectodomain shedding. FASEB J. 2010;24:916–930. DOI: 10.1096/fj.09-140921

[122] Stattin P, Björ O, Ferrari P, Lukanova A, Lenner P, Lindhal B, Hallmans G, Kaaks R: Prospective study of hyperglycemia and cancer risk. Diabetes Care. 2007;30:561–567.

[123] Abe R, Shimizu T, Sugawara H, Watanabe H, Nakamura H, Choei H, Sasaki N, Yamagishi S, Takeuchi M, Shimizu H: Regulation of human melanoma growth and metastasis by AGE-AGR receptor interactions. J Invest Dermatol. 2004;122:461–467.

[124] Takeuchi M, Samagishi S: TAGE (toxic AGEs) hypothesis in various chronic diseases. Med Hypoth. 2004;63:449–452.

[125] Ojima A, Matsui T, Maeda S, Takeuchi M, Inoue H, Higashimoto Y, Yamagishi SI: DNA aptamer raised against advanced glycation end products inhibits melanoma growth in nude mice. Lab Invest. 2014;94:422–429. DOI: 10.1038/labinvest.2014.5

[126] Meghnani V, Vetter SW, Leclerc E: RAGE overexpression confers a metastatic phenotype of the WM115 human primary melanoma cell line. Biochim Biophys Acta. 2014;1842;1017–1027. DOI: 10.1016/j.bbadis.2014.02.01

[127] Mizumoto S, Sugahara K: Glycosaminoglycans are functional ligands for receptor for advanced glycation end-product in tumors. FEBS J. 2012;280:2462–2470. DOI: 10.1111/febs.12156

[128] Saha A, Lee YC, Zhang Z, Chandra G, Su SB, Makherjee AB: Lack of an endogenous anti-inflammatory protein in mice enhances colonization of B16F10 melanoma cell in the lungs. J Biol Chem. 2010;285:10822–10831. DOI: 10.1074/jbc.M109.083550

[129] Hofmann MA, Drury S, Fu C, Qu W, Taguchi A, Lu Y, Avila C, Kambham N, Bierhaus A, Nawroth P, Neurath MF, Slattery T, Beach D, McClary J, Nagashima M, Morser J, Stern D, Schmidt MA: RAGE mediates a novel proinflamatory axis: a central cell surface receptor for S100/calgranulin polypeptides. Cell. 1999;97:889–901.

[130] Salama I, Malone PS, Mihaimeed F, Jones JL: A review of the S100 proteins in cancer. EJSO. 2008;34:357–364. DOI: 10.1016/j.ejso.2007.04.009

[131] Ugurel S, Utikal J, Becker JC: Tumor biomarkers in melanoma. Cancer Control. 2009;16:219–224.

[132] Weide B, Elsasser M, Büttner P, Pflugfelder A, Leiter U, Eigentler TK, Bauer J, Witte M, Meier F, Garbe C: Serum markers lactate dehydrogenase and S100B predict independently disease outcome in melanoma patients with distant metastasis. Br J Cancer. 2012;107:422–428. DOI: 10.1038/bjc.2012.306

[133] Gebhardt C, Lichtenberger R, Utikal J: Biomarker value and pitfalls of serum S100B in the follow-up of high-risk melanoma patients. J Dtsch Dermatol Ges. 2016;14:158–164. DOI: 10.1111/ddg.12727

[134] Wagner NB, Weide B, Reith M, Tarnanidis K, Kehrel C, Lichtenberger R, Pflugfelder A, Herpel E, Eubel J, Ikenberg K, Busch C, Holland-Letz T, Naeher H, Garbe C, Umansky V, Enk A, Utikal J, Gebhardt C: Diminished levels of the soluble form of RAGE are related to poor survival in malignant melanoma. Int J Cancer. 2015;137:2607–2617. DOI: 10.1002/ijc.29619

[135] Yoshimura C, Miyafusa T, Tsumoto K: Identification of small-molecule inhibitors of the human S100B-p53 interaction and evaluation of their activity in human melanoma cells. Bioorg Med Chem. 2013;21:1109–1115. DOI: 10.1016/j.bmc.2012.12.042

[136] Zimmer DB, Lapidus RG, Weber DJ: In vivo screening of S100B inhibitors for melanoma therapy. Methods Mol Biol. 2013;963:303–317. DOI: 10.1007/978-1-62703-230-8_18

[137] Zhu L, Ito T, Nakahara T, Nagae K, Fuyuno Y, Nakao M, Akahoshi M, Nakagawa R, Tu Y, Uchi H, Furue M: Upregulation of S100P, receptor for advanced glycation end products and ezrin in malignant melanoma. J Dermatol. 2013;40:973–979. DOI: 10.1111/1346-8138.12323

[138] Wang G, Platt-Higgins A, Carroll J, de Silva Rudland S, Winstanley J, Barraclough R, Rudland PS: Induction of metastasis by S100P in a rat mammary model and its association with poor survival of breast cancer patients. Cancer Res. 2006;66:1199–1207.

Chapter 5

Cadherins and their Role in Malignant Transformation: Implications for Skin Cancer Progression

Marcelina E. Janik, Dorota Hoja-Łukowicz and
Małgorzata Przybyło

Additional information is available at the end of the chapter

http://dx.doi.org/10.5772/64666

Abstract

Cadherins are a large family of Ca^{2+}dependent adhesion proteins. They are transmembrane or closely related to membrane glycoproteins localized in specialized adhesive junction. The expression of various cadherins may be concomitant with cancer progression steps and the term 'cadherin switch' has been created due to the observation of down-regulation of E-cadherin (suppressor of metastatic potential) and up-regulation of N-cadherin (promoter of metastatic potential) expression during tumour progression. These changes are thought to be closely related to epithelial-to-mesenchymal transition of cells of many different types of cancer including skin cancers, and accompany the increase of their motility and invasion abilities resulting in the metastasis formation. The cadherin polypeptide is a potential substrate for post-translational modification, for example, N-glycosylation, and its important role in the regulation of cadherin function has been described. The changed glycosylation of cadherins has been described in various skin cancers including melanoma and was consistent with cadherins' role in epithelial-to-mesenchymal transition. The detailed analysis of cadherin expression and cadherin-related glycosylation changes taking place during malignant transformation could be a key for better understanding of the nature of this process and may open new opportunities for the creation of more effective anticancer therapeutics and diagnostic tools.

Keywords: cadherins, melanoma, basal cell carcinoma, squamous cell carcinoma, glycosylation, metastasis

1. Introduction

In humans, cadherins comprise a superfamily of over 100 calcium-dependent adhesion molecules that play fundamental roles in supervising morphogenetic and differentiation processes during development, and in maintaining tissue architecture and homeostasis [1]. Therefore, their expression is tightly regulated during development, and abnormalities in the expression or function of cadherins are characteristic features of transformed cells. Being transmembrane proteins, cadherins are built from extracellular, transmembranous and cytoplasmic domains. The only exception is an unusual T (truncated)-cadherin, which is similar to the classical cadherins in terms of ectodomain construction, but differs from them by lacking both the transmembrane and cytoplasmic domains. Instead, T-cadherin is linked to plasma membrane through a glycosylphosphatidylinositol (GPI) anchor [2]. Extracellular domain of T-cadherin lacks many amino acids, which are responsible for the adhesive function of the classical cadherins. Therefore, it is suggested that T-cadherin functions as a signalling molecule rather than as a cell adhesion molecule [3].

According to the sequence similarity, cadherins have been divided into five subfamilies: classical types I and II (E-, P-, N- and VE-cadherin), atypical (T-cadherin), desmosomal (desmogleins, desmocollins), protocadherins and cadherin-related proteins [4]. Cadherins maintain stable cell-cell adhesion via homophilic interactions of their extracellular regions that trigger the assembly of specialized adhesive junctions (AJs) known as desmosomes and adherens junctions, and tethering the microfilaments and intermediated filaments to the plasma membrane by the cytoplasmic domains [5]. In this way, cadherins, by mediating adhesion, provide a cohesion and communication between cells in a tissue [1]. The cytoplasmic region anchors cadherin to actin cytoskeleton via interaction with catenin family—β-catenin, γ-catenin, which binds directly to cadherin tail, and α-catenin, which links β- or γ-catenin to actin.

β-catenin is attached to cadherin in the endoplasmic reticulum at the early stage of its targeting to the plasma membrane, where they are present as a complex. Therefore, this cadherin-β-catenin interaction is independent of cadherin engagement in adhesion [6]. α-catenin has been perceived as a constituent stably binding the β-catenin-cadherin complex to actin cytoskeleton, but it has been shown nowadays that allosteric character of α-catenin indisposes its binding to β-catenin and F-actin at the same time [7]. Another member of the catenin family, p120-catenin, attaches to the cadherin-catenin complex in the plasma membrane and controls cadherin turnover by stabilization of the complex assembly at the plasma membrane. p120-catenin knockdown experiments with the use of RNAi have shown a more rapid turnover and degradation of cadherin complexes [8]. β-catenin and p120-catenin are substrates of tyrosine kinase receptor, and therefore the adhesion could be regulated by the action of growth factors [9]. Clustering of AJs results in remodelling of the actin cytoskeleton [10–13]. There is a wide variety of proteins associated with cadherins and this association is thought to be transient and adjustable dependent on cell context and the triggered cellular-signalling pathways [14].

First reports of Ca^{2+}-dependent surface glycoproteins mediating intercellular adhesion have regarded chick development and process of morula compaction in pre-implantation mouse

http://dx.doi.org/10.5772/64666

embryo [15–18]. The first identified, E-cadherin is a classical type I cadherin, and its prefix 'E' refers to the epithelial cells (ECs) where it was originally described. Other classical cadherins of a different spatiotemporal expression pattern include N-cadherin (neural, type I), P-cadherin (placenta, type I) [19], R-cadherin (retina, type I) [20] and VE-cadherin (vascular endothelial, type II) [21].

The structure of classic cadherin molecules is more or less conserved; they possess a cytoplasmic domain associated with the armadillo proteins family [22], and in the case of E-cadherin this region comprises 150 aa [4]. Next, there is a single-pass transmembrane region, and extracellular domain of 550 aa, which in classic cadherins (types I and II), desmosomal and T-cadherin contain five segments of a repeated sequence. The extracellular domains are numbered from EC1 to EC5, where the sequence of the headmost EC5 is characteristic because of the presence of four conserved cysteine residues [4, 23, 24]. In the extracellular domain between the adjacent EC domains, the highly conserved Ca^{2+}-binding sequences are located.

Based on E-cadherin structure analysis, several possible mechanisms of cadherin-mediated cell-cell adhesion have been proposed. Cadherins could form either *trans* dimers, where the linkage is formed by cadherins from apposed cells, or *cis* dimers, where the lateral interaction between cadherin molecules in the same cell membrane takes place. Their formation depends on Ca^{2+} availability. In Ca^{2+} presence, *trans* dimers are formed preferentially, while in its absence *cis* dimer formation predominates. Furthermore, *trans* dimers are thought to be responsible for cell-cell adhesion, and the formation of *cis* dimers has been reported to enhance the strength of adhesive interaction [11, 25]. Both dimers are formed via the same region of cadherin molecules—EC1 domain; however, the involvement of EC3 domain has also been confirmed in the case of *trans* dimerization process. Concerning EC1 and EC3 role in *trans* dimerization, three possible adhesive antiparallel alignments have been proposed, starting from the outermost adhesive bonds between EC1 domains, through middle bond requiring both EC1 and EC3 contribution in bond formation, and finally the innermost adhesive bounds formed by the EC3 domains [26]. The classic model assumed that there are homophilic interactions between cadherins, but growing evidence suggests also the presence of heterophilic ones. Shan and co-workers have reported heterophilic interactions between R- and N-cadherins interacting either in *cis* or in *trans* manner [25]. Importantly, cadherins can be post-translationally modified by phosphorylation, O-glycosylation but the most prominent modification is N-glycosylation [10, 27–29].

2. Cadherins and skin cancers

It is well known that the transformation of normal tissue cells to tumour cells is associated with the changes in the repertoire of cell-surface adhesions, such as cadherins, and carbohydrate structures are attached to them. Altered glycosylated cell-surface glycoproteins influence the growth, proliferation and survival of tumour cells, and facilitate their migratory and invasion behaviour, formation of distant metastases as well as the induction of immunosuppression. It is noteworthy that tumour-associated antigens can serve as valuable diagnostic and therapeutic targets.

Skin tumours comprise melanoma and non-melanoma skin cancers. Non-melanoma neoplasms are mainly divided into basal cell carcinoma (BCC), squamous cell carcinoma (SCC), keratoacanthoma (KA, a benign low-grade skin tumour without the competence to metastasize or invade), trichoepithelioma (TE, a benign skin tumour, which arises from the hair germ), actinic keratosis (AK, a precancerous stage of squamous cell carcinoma) and Merkel cell carcinoma (MCC, an early metastasizing neoplasm of high-grade malignancy). Although melanoma is much less common, it possesses high potential to invade surrounding tissues and very quickly develops distant metastases. Therefore, melanoma is the leading cause of deaths from skin cancer.

2.1. Cadherins in the skin

In human skin, the expression of several cadherin molecules, belonging to all five major groups of the cadherin family, has been described. The changes in their protein levels have been extensively investigated regarding the developmental processes and neoplastic transformation of skin cells (**Table 1**). The vast majority of research studies concern classical cadherins. Both E- and P-cadherins are the major components of the intercellular AJs of the epidermis [30], and they are main players in morphogenesis and in maintaining the structure of the skin. Referring to E-cadherin, the wide distribution of its expression in all skin layers and in skin appendages has been shown, and its role in keratinocytes-melanocytes adhesion and communication has been established. It has been reported that E- and N-cadherin-negative dermal stem cells (DSCs), isolated from human foreskin dermis during their differentiation into melanocytes and migration to the epidermis, gain E-cadherin expression, enabling them to interact with the keratinocytes [31]. On the other hand, *in vitro* experiments in melanocytes and keratinocytes co-cultures have shown that during wound healing and re-pigmentation process, diminished E-cadherin expression in melanocytes increases their migration capacity as they migrate much faster than keratinocytes into the wound area [32].

The expression of P-cadherin, which is known to be indispensable for proper skin and eye function, has been more diversified and dependent on the skin layer. It is mainly present in the basal and lower suprabasal layers, where it was linked with the proliferative compartment of the epidermis. The predominant expression of P-cadherin has also been observed in the growing hair follicle, where it has an important role in its differentiation. Moreover, P-cadherin has been suggested to have a regulatory effect on melanogenesis, mainly due to the inhibition of tyrosinase activity, and to regulate melanosome transport within the melanosome unit [24].

The expression of N-cadherin has also been described in the skin during developmental processes, referring to dermal fibroblasts and endothelial cells but not in keratinocytes or melanocytes [33]. N-cadherin expression has been analysed in murine model of melanocytes development and *in vitro* cultured melanoblast, melanocyte and melanoma cell lines. The melanoblasts/melanocytes of a 3-day-old mouse dermis have expressed only small amount of N-cadherin, while its significantly higher expression has been reported in all *in vitro* models [34]. The changed expression of N-cadherin on dermal melanocytes has been suggested to enable their migration during developmental processes and stabilized their interaction with dermal fibroblasts [35].

Type I classical cadherins

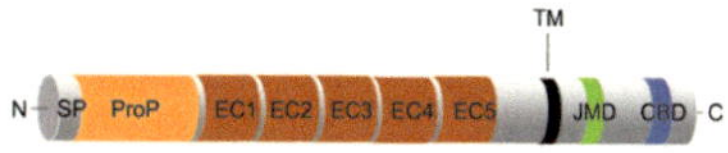

Protein	Gen (location)	Protein expression level in cancer skin tissue[a]		Structure[b]
Cadherin 1 (E-cadherin)	*CDH1* (16q22.1)	K: 100; BCC: 23 / 57 / 20; SCC: 7 / 59 / 24 / 4	M: 100; Melanoma: 10 / 40 / 13 / 37	E-cadherin
Cadherin 2 (N-cadherin)	*CDH2* (18q12.1)	K: 100; BCC: 8 / 92; SCC: 100	M: 100; Melanoma: 13 / 6 / 10 / 71	
Cadherin-3 (P-cadherin)	*CDH3* (16q22.1)	K: 100; BCC: 18 / 82; SCC: 10 / 90	M: 100; Melanoma: 32 / 37 / 26 / 5	
Cadherin 4 (R-cadherin)	*CDH4* (20q13.33)	K: 100; BCC: 100; SCC: 86 / 14	M: 100; Melanoma: 17 / 25 / 58	

Type II classical cadherins

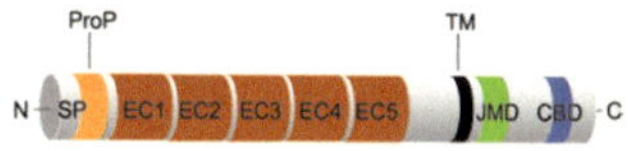

Protein	Gen (location)	Protein expression level in cancer skin tissue[a]		Structure[b]
Cadherin 5 (VE-cadherin)	*CDH5* (16q21)	K: 100; BCC: 60 / 40; SCC: 50 / 50	M: 100; Melanoma: 83 / 17	cadherin 11
Cadherin 6 (K-cadherin)	*CDH6* (5p13.3)	K: 100; BCC: 47 / 53; SCC: 10.5 / 63 / 26,5	M: 100; Melanoma: 9 / 91	
Cadherin 7	*CDH7* (18q22.1)	K: 100; BCC: 100; SCC: 100	M: 100; Melanoma: 9 / 91	
Cadherin 9 (T1-cadherin)	*CDH9* (5p14.1)	K: 100; BCC: 20 / 80; SCC: 83 / 17	M: 100; Melanoma: 25 / 67 / 8	
Cadherin 11 (OB-cadherin)	*CDH11* (16q21)	K: 100; BCC: 75 / 25; SCC: 100	M: 100; Melanoma: 17 / 83	
Cadherin 12 (N-cadherin 2)	*CDH12* (5p14.3)	K: 100; BCC: 50 / 50; SCC: 17 / 50 / 33	M: 100; Melanoma: 33 / 33 / 34	
Cadherin 18	*CDH18* (5p14.3)	K: 100; BCC: 100; SCC: 100	M: 100; Melanoma: 27 / 27 / 46	
Cadherin 19	*CDH19* (18q22.1)	K: 100; BCC: 100; SCC: 12,5 / 87,5	M: 100; Melanoma: 8 / 92	
Cadherin 20	*CDH20* (18q21.33)	K: 100; BCC: 100; SCC: 43 / 57	M: 100; Melanoma: 50 / 42 / 8	
Cadherin 22	*CDH22* (20q13.12)	K: 100; BCC: 100; SCC: 14 / 86	M: 100; Melanoma: 27 / 27 / 46	

Truncated/atypical cadherin

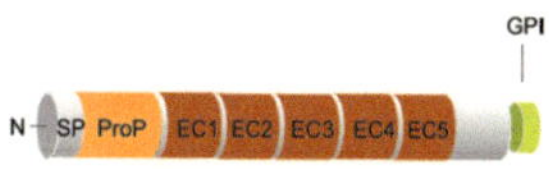

Protein	Gen (location)	Protein expression level in cancer skin tissue[a]		Structure[b]
Cadherin 13 (H-cadherin, T-cadherin)	*CDH13* (16q23.3)	K: 100; BCC: 23 / 73; SCC: 8 / 92	M: 100; Melanoma: 100	T-cadherin

Protein	Gen (location)	Protein expression level in cancer skin tissue[a]		Structure[b]
Desmosomal cadherins				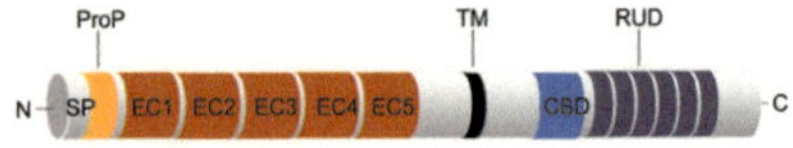
Desmoglein 1	*DSG1* (18q12.1)	K: 100; BCC: 9 / 27 / 64; SCC: 18 / 55 / 18 / 9	M: 100; Melanoma: 17 / 83	Desmoglein 2
Desmoglein 2	*DSG2* (18q12.1)	K: 100; BCC: 18 / 73 / 9; SCC: 18 / 82	M: 100; Melanoma: 100	
Desmoglein 3	*DSG3* (18q12.1)	K: 100; BCC: 15 / 85; SCC: 44 / 19 / 37	M: 100; Melanoma: 100	
Desmoglein 4	*DSG4* (18q12.1)	K: 100; BCC: 20 / 80; SCC: 14 / 86	M: 100; Melanoma: 100	
Desmocollin 1	*DSC1* (18q12.1)	K: 100; BCC: 100; SCC: 29 / 29 / 42	M: 100; Melanoma: 67 / 33	
Desmocollin 2	*DSC2* (18q12.1)	K: 100; BCC: 75 / 25; SCC: 71 / 29	M: 100; Melanoma: 9 / 91	
Desmocollin 3	*DSC3* (18q12.1)	K: 100; BCC: 10 / 20 / 50 / 20; SCC: 36.5 / 36.5 / 9 / 18	M: 100; Melanoma: 100	
Protocadherins clustered				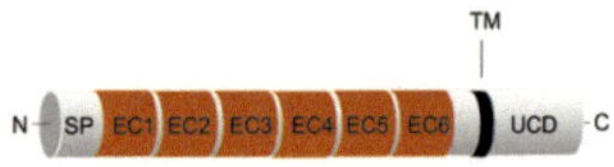
Protocadherin α 1	*PCDHA1* (5q31.3)	K: 100; BCC: 100; SCC: 100	M: 100; Melanoma: 9 / 91	Protocadherin β 1
Protocadherin α 2	*PCDHA2* (5q31.3)	K: 100; BCC: 100; SCC: 17 / 33 / 50	M: 100; Melanoma: 55 / 27 / 18	
Protocadherin α 3	*PCDHA3* (5q31.3)	K: 100; BCC: 100; SCC: 100	M: 100; Melanoma: 67 / 33	
Protocadherin α 5	*PCDHA5* (5q31.3)	K: 100; BCC: 100; SCC: 8 / 92	M: 100; Melanoma: 16 / 42 / 42	
Protocadherin α 8	*PCDHA8* (5q31.3)	K: 100; BCC: 100; SCC: 100	M: 100; Melanoma: 100	
Protocadherin α 12	*PCDHA12* (5q31.3)	K: 100; BCC: 100; SCC: 8 / 92	M: 100; Melanoma: 8 / 8 / 84	
Protocadherin β 1	*PCDHB1* (5q31.3)	K: 100; BCC: 25 / 75; SCC: 43 / 57	M: 100; Melanoma: 42 / 58	
Protocadherin β 2	*PCDHB2* (5q31.3)	K: 100; BCC: 100; SCC: 100	M: 100; Melanoma: 8 / 92	
Protocadherin β 3	*PCDHB3* (5q31.3)	K: 100; BCC: 100; SCC: 100	M: 100; Melanoma: 100	
Protocadherin β4	*PCDHB4* (5q31.3)	K: 100; BCC: 20 / 80; SCC: 100	M: 100; Melanoma: 42 / 58	

Protein	Gen (location)	Protein expression level in cancer skin tissue[a]		Structure[b]
Protocadherin β 5	*PCDHB5* (5q31.3)	K: 100; BCC: 100; SCC: 9, 91	M: 100; Melanoma: 33, 50, 27	
Protocadherin β 6	*PCDHB6* (5q31.3)	K: 100; BCC: 20, 80; SCC: 14, 86	M: 100; Melanoma: 25, 75	
Protocadherin β 7	*PCDHB7* (5q31.3)	K: 100; BCC: 100; SCC: 2.5, 75, 12.5	M: 100; Melanoma: 12.5, 50, 37.5	
Protocadherin β 8	*PCDHB8* (5q31.3)	K: 100; BCC: 100; SCC: 100	M: 100; Melanoma: 18, 64, 18	
Protocadherin β 9/10	*PCDHB9/10* (5q31.3)	K: 100; BCC: 30, 40, 30; SCC: 28.5, 50, 21.5	M: 100; Melanoma: 17, 50, 33	
Protocadherin β 11/12	*PCDHB11/12* (5q31.3)	K: 100; BCC: 50, 50; SCC: 50, 50	M: 100; Melanoma: 83, 17	
Protocadherin β 14	*PCDHB14* (5q31.3)	K: 100; BCC: 33, 67; SCC: 100	M: 100; Melanoma: 17, 83	
Protocadherin β 15	*PCDHB15* (5q31.3)	K: 100; BCC: 30, 20, 50; SCC: 25, 33, 42	M: 100; Melanoma: 10, 90	
Protocadherin γ subfamily A, 1	*PCDHGA1* (5q31.3)	K: 100; BCC: 40, 60; SCC: 17, 83	M: 100; Melanoma: 18, 64, 9, 9	
Protocadherin γ subfamily B, 3	*PCDHGB3* (5q31.3)	K: 100; BCC: 33, 67; SCC: 67, 33	M: 100; Melanoma: 8, 25, 67	
Protocadherins nonclustered δ1				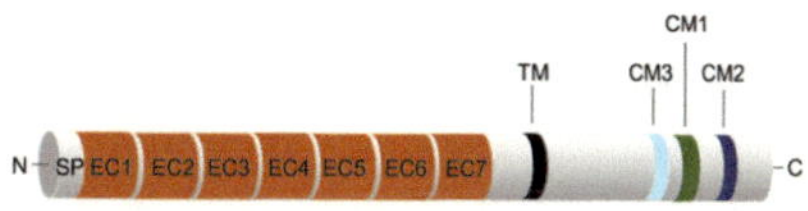
Protocadherin 1	*PCDH1* (5q31.3)	K: 100; BCC: 43, 57; SCC: 44, 12, 44	M: 100; Melanoma: 45.5, 54.5	Protocadherin 1
Protocadherin 7	*PCDH7* (4p15.1)	K: 100; BCC: 100; SCC: 43, 43, 14	M: 100; Melanoma: 27, 64, 9	
Protocadherin 9	*PCDH9* (13q21.32)	K: 100; BCC: 100; SCC: 100	M: 100; Melanoma: 8, 17, 75	
Protocadherin 11 X/Y-linked	*PCDH11X/Y* (Xq21.31/ Yp11.2)	K: 100; BCC: 100; SCC: 17, 83	M: 100; Melanoma: 8, 25, 67	
Protocadherins nonclustered δ2				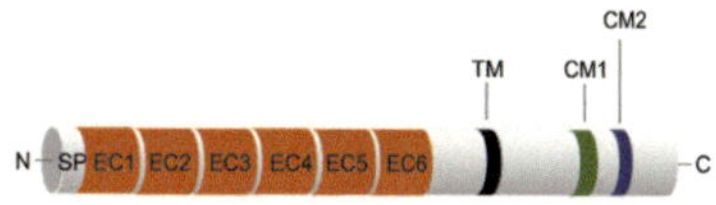
Protocadherin 8	*PCDH8* (13q14.3)	K: 100; BCC: 25, 25, 50; SCC: 17, 17, 66	M: 100; Melanoma: 46, 27, 27	Protocadherin 8
Protocadherin 10	*PCDH10* (4q28.3)	K: 100; BCC: 25, 50, 25; SCC: 100	M: 100; Melanoma: 17, 42, 41	

Protein	Gen (location)	Protein expression level in cancer skin tissue[a]		Structure[b]
Protocadherin 17	*PCDH17* (13q21.1)	K: 100; BCC: 20, 60, 20; SCC: 43, 28.5, 28.5	M: 100; Melanoma: 17, 50, 33	
Protocadherin 18	*PCDH18* (4q28.3)	K: 100; BCC: 40, 60; SCC: 57, 43	M: 100; Melanoma: 58, 42	
Protocadherin 19	*PCDH19* (Xq22.1)	K: 100; BCC: 100; SCC: 100	M: 100; Melanoma: 8, 8, 84	
Cadherin-releted proteins				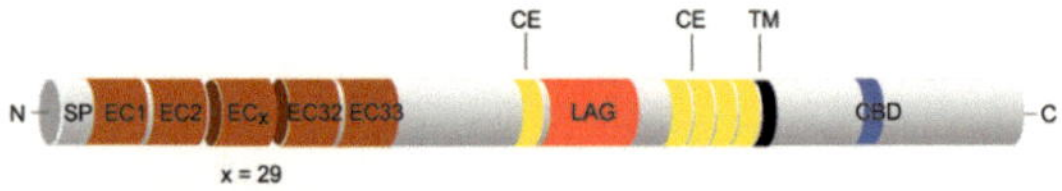
Cadherin-related 23	*CDH23* (10q22.1)	K: 100; BCC: 66, 34; SCC: 33, 33, 34	M: 100; Melanoma: 9, 73, 18	FAT atypical cadherin 1
Dachsous cadherin-related 1	*DCHS1* (11p15.4)	K: 100; BCC: 44, 44, 12; SCC: 8, 92	M: 100; Melanoma: 90, 10	
Dachsous cadherin-related 2	*DCHS2* (4q31.3)	K: 100; BCC: 40, 40, 20; SCC: 100	M: 100; Melanoma: 58, 8, 17, 17	
Cadherin 26	*CDH26* (20q13.33)	K: 100; BCC: 100; SCC: 100	M: 100; Melanoma: 8, 92	
Cadherin-related family member 1	*CDHR1* (10q23.1)	K: 100; BCC: 100; SCC: 14, 86	M: 100; Melanoma: 27, 73	
Cadherin-related family member 2	*CDHR2* (5q35.2)	K: 100; BCC: 100; SCC: 100	M: 100; Melanoma: 100	
Cadherin-related family member 4	*CDHR4* (3p21.31)	K: 100; BCC: 17, 33, 50; SCC: 17, 17, 59, 16	M: 100; Melanoma: 92, 8	
Protocadherin 12 (VE-cadherin-2)	*PCDH12* (5q31.3)	K: 100; BCC: 100; SCC: 14, 86	M: 100; Melanoma: 36, 36, 28	
FAT atypical cadherin 1	*FAT1* (4q35.2)	K: 100; BCC: 58, 42; SCC: 18, 46, 36	M: 100; Melanoma: 44, 44, 12	
FAT atypical cadherin 3	*FAT3* (11q14.3)	K: 100; BCC: 100; SCC: 83, 17	M: 100; Melanoma: 100	
FAT atypical cadherin 4	*FAT4* (4q28.1)	K: 100; BCC: 100; SCC: 17, 83	M: 100; Melanoma: 27, 73	
Calsyntenin 1	*CLSTN1* 1 p36.22)	K: 100; BCC: 60, 40; SCC: 14, 86	M: 100; Melanoma: 36, 27, 27, 10	
Calsyntenin 2	*CLSTN2* (3q23)	K: 100; BCC: 60, 40; SCC: 14, 86	M: 100; Melanoma: 11, 89	
Calsyntenin 3	*CLSTN 3* (12p13.31)	K: 100; BCC: 33, 67; SCC: 37.5, 62.5	M: 100; Melanoma: 8, 17, 17, 58	
Ret proto-oncogene	*CRET* (10q11.21)	K: 100; BCC: 37, 25, 19, 19; SCC: 33, 11, 23, 33	M: 100; Melanoma: 33, 87	

http://dx.doi.org/10.5772/64666

Protein	Gen (location)	Protein expression level in cancer skin tissue[a]		Structure[b]
Cadherin, EGF LAG seven-pass G-type receptor 2	*CELSR2* (1p13.3)	K: 100 BCC: 100 SCC: 37.5 / 50 / 12.5	M: 100 Melanoma: 8 / 67 / 25	
Cadherin, EGF LAG seven-pass G-type receptor 3	*CELSR3* (3p21.31)	K: 100 BCC: 20 / 40 / 40 SCC: 33 / 50 / 17	M: 100 Melanoma: 33 / 58 / 9	

[a]Antibody staining/cadherin expression level in human keratinocytes, BCC, SCC and in human melanocytes and melanoma cells, respectively, described by the colour-coding scales: ■/■ high, ■/■ medium, ■/■ low, □/□ not detected. The numbers within bars correspond to the percentage of a given staining/cadherin expression level. Data for protocadherins γ 2-12 of subfamily A, protocadherins γ 1,2,4-7 of subfamily B and protocadherins γ 3-5 of subfamily C have not been analysed due to the antibodies that cross-reacted with multiple isoforms. Data are based on The Human Protein Atlas (www.proteinatlas.org).

[b]Schematic structure of a representative member of the given cadherin subfamily.

BCC, basal cell carcinoma; K, keratinocyte; M, melanocyte; and SCC, squamous cell carcinoma; C, COOH terminus of protein; CBD, β-catenin-binding domain or plakoglobin-binding domain in the case of desmosomal cadherins; CE, cysteine-rich EGF-repeat-like domain; CM1-3, conserved motifs in the cytoplasmic domains of nonclustered δ-protocadherins; EC, extracellular cadherin repeats; GPI, glycosylphosphatidylinositol anchor; JMD, juxtamembrane domain with p120-catenin-binding site; LAG, laminin-A globular domain-like domain; N, NH_2-terminus of protein; ProP, propeptide; RUD, intracellular repeated unit domain of desmosomal cadherins; SP, signal peptide; TM, transmembrane domain; and UCD, unique cytoplasmic domain.

Table 1. Comparison of the expression pattern of cadherins in keratinocytes versus BCCs and SCCs, and melanocytes versus melanoma cells.

In normal skin, the expression of T-cadherin is mostly limited to melanocytes and actively proliferating keratinocytes of the basal layer, as well as to a lesser extent to dermal blood vessels. Unlike other cadherins, T-cadherin molecules are anchored in lipid rafts dispersed on the whole cell plasma membrane [36].

The changes in the expression level of particular cadherins, named 'cadherin switch', concerning the down-regulation of E-cadherin expression mediating strong adhesion signal, and recognized as an invasion suppressor, and the up-regulation of N-cadherin expression inducing more motile and invasive phenotype of cells have been suggested either during development or in cancer, where it may be concomitant with cancer progression steps [37–39]. The 'cadherin switch' has been observed and described as an indispensable step, enabling the epithelial-to-mesenchymal transition (EMT).

2.2. Role of cadherins in epithelial-to-mesenchymal transition

EMT is a process of dedifferentiation, which has been described by three major cell phenotype changes, including (1) diminution of cellular adhesion, as an effect of changes in the expression of adhesion receptors and cytoskeletal proteins; (2) loss of epithelial cell polarity accompanied by morphological changes leading from the cobblestone-like epithelial cells to spindle-shaped mesenchymal cells; and (3) the acquisition of more motile and invasive behaviour [40, 41]. This process takes place during normal embryonic development as a basic step of tissue remodelling, such as mesoderm formation and neural crest development. It should be noted that the reverse process, named mesenchymal-to-epithelial transition (MET), also occurs evidencing the enormous plasticity of developmental processes [40]. EMT-like processes are observed also in the course of wound healing, during which in response to injury keratinocytes go through a 'metastable' phenotype by losing their contact and therefore move [42]. EMT has been suggested in numerous cancer types, including melanoma and supposed as a conducive to metastasis formation.

2.2.1. *EMT molecular markers*

Besides or as a consequence of EMT-related 'cadherin switch', more abundant expression of vimentin with simultaneous β-catenin translocation to the nucleus, and increased expression of transcription factors such as Slug, Snail, Twist, EF1/ZEB1, SIP1/ZEB2 and E47 have been observed. They are reported as markers of developmental processes [43–45] and skin cancer cells transformation [38, 46, 47]. It is noteworthy that the suggestion is made on the basis of metastatic BCC observations that the enhanced Twist1 expression may serve as a biomarker of BCC progression [48]. Immunohistochemical analysis of tissue sections of non-metastasizing, metastasizing and lymph node metastasis of cutaneous SCC (cSCC) has revealed that their metastatic potential is accompanied by EMT-marker expression, including the Twist overexpression, while in metastases the expression of selected EMT-related markers has been decreased [49]. Also, the increased expression of other EMT-related markers such as Ki-67 and keratin 17, together with the reduced expression of both E-cadherin and involucrin (early marker of epidermis keratinocytes differentiation), has been shown in the cSCC compared to normal skin biopsies [50].

Some studies suggested that the EMT is closely related with the cancer stem cells (CSCs) biology, and therefore the analysis of expression of CD44 and CD29 (β1-integrin subunit) recognized as CSCs markers has been conducted in cSCC A341 cells. High expression of both markers has been described in cells located in the periphery of cSCC tumours. Simultaneously, a higher N-cadherin and a lower E-cadherin expression have been detected in CD44+/CD29+ cells, legitimizing their EMT [51]. In human, BCC analysis of paraffin-embedded tissue sections suggested strong correlation between tumour progression and the expression of integrin-linked kinase (ILK), which has been proposed there as an EMT marker [52].

The expression of EMT markers has been analysed in desmoplastic melanoma (DM) tumours, which makes diagnostic difficulties because of its unusual clinical appearance. These are mainly amelanotic, deep cutaneous tumours surrounded by sun-damaged skin [53]. The comparison of EMT markers expression profile conducted in tissue microarrays of DM and primary vertical growth phase non-desmoplastic melanomas (NDMs) has demonstrated a significantly higher expression of EMT-related proteins—N-cadherin, SPARC and WT-1, and the decreased expression of E-cadherin in DM compared to NDM, suggesting usefulness of these markers in DM diagnostics [54].

Another known marker of EMT and tumour metastasis is the elevated expression of N-acetylglucosaminyltransferase V (GnT-V) responsible for β1,6-branching of N-linked complex-type oligosaccharides. In cutaneous wound healing of GnT-V transgenic mice, GnT-V-overexpressed keratinocytes showed spindle-shaped morphology and enhanced migration, which were associated with the early phase of malignant transformation: changes in E-cadherin glycosylation and localization as well as induction of EMT. As a result, EMT-associated factors Snail and Twist were up-regulated, and cadherin switch was observed [55].

2.2.2. *EMT-initiating factors*

EMT initiation has been attributed to a variety of growth factors, including members of the epidermal growth factor (EGF), the fibroblast growth factor (FGF) and the insulin-like growth factor (IGF) families, hepatocyte growth factor (HGF) and transforming growth factor-β (TGF-β). The intracellular-signalling pathways, induced by these growth factors, have led to characteristic transformation from epithelial, differentiated and proliferative phenotype to mesenchymal, dedifferentiated ready to migration and invasion phenotype. Down-regulated dermal fibroblast secretion of HGF caused by knockdown of RalA GTPase expression (known contributor in Ras-induced tumourigenesis) has resulted in the suppression of SCC tumour progression. As an effect, the reduced migratory abilities of neighbouring keratinocytes, related to the changes in expression levels of E-cadherin (increased) and transcription factors —Snail and Slug—suppressing E-cadherin RNA level, have been observed [56]. The TGF-β-induced EMT has been observed in melanoma cells and accompanied by the activation of the PI3K and platelet-derived growth factor (PDGF)-signalling pathways triggering the up-regulation of N-cadherin expression and the transformation of a proliferative phenotype of cells into a more invasive one [57].

The involvement of PI3K/AKT-signalling pathway has also been suggested in EMT of SCC cells. The analysis of isogenic cell lines derived from succeeding stages of keratinocytes malignant transformation, that is, dysplastic forehead skin (PM1), primary cSCC (MET1) and its lymph node metastasis (MET4), has shown the correlation between tumour progression and the activation of AKT. Additionally, it has been reported that the inhibition of AKT activity results in the decreased cell migration and invasion, reduced cell detachment and reduced expression of EMT markers such as Slug and vimentin concomitantly with the up-regulation of E-cadherin expression [46].

There are also some data concerning the relevance of cytokine IL-6 secretion during the inflammatory processes for the initiation of EMT and subsequent malignant transformation of normal human keratinocytes of HaCat cell line. In response to arsenite treatment, the elevated IL-6 secretion has been observed leading to the increased level of miR-21, microRNA related with the malignancies and overexpressed in most cancers. The arsenite-transformed HaCat cells have shown the changed expression level of E-cadherin (decreased) and vimentin (increased), which was linked with the initiation of EMT process and increased migration capacity of transformed cells [58]. As melanoma patients are characterized by a higher IL-6 serum level, its important role in the stimulation of melanoma progression has been suggested.

In a mouse melanoma model, the action of IL-6 has led to the increased metastatic potential due to up-regulation of Twist expression and subsequent N-cadherin overexpression. Thus, therapies directed specifically against IL-6 could possibly reduce the tumour progression [59].

In response to mechanical tissue damage, and succeeding action of cytokines and growth factors (TGF-β, EGF), the activation of specific signalling pathways has been reported in skin keratinocytes, leading to the activation of Snail—a regulator of keratinocytes inflammatory response and an EMT marker. Snail protein acts as gene transcription repressors, and E-cadherin gene has been recognized as its prototypic target. Down-regulated E-cadherin expression facilitates the process of wound healing by losing adhesion between keratinocytes, EMT promotion and subsequent keratinocyte migration. Likewise, in the course of keratinocyte neoplastic transformation, signalling via Snail promotes migration and invasion phenotype, proinflammatory microenvironment and degradation of extracellular matrix characteristic for SCC [60]. These processes are similar in many carcinoma types and suggestion has been made that tumours resemble wounds that do not heal [61].

2.3. Cancer-related changes in cadherin expression

While the neoplastic transformation of many cell types is accompanied by the loss of or disturbances in gap junction formation, the neoplastic transformation of melanocytes and keratinocytes follows the same path. It has been observed that the diminished E-cadherin expression level, typical for melanoma cells, disturbs their interaction with adjacent keratinocytes and therefore prevents the regulating influence of keratinocytes on the melanoma cells growth and differentiation [62]. The large body of evidence has suggested that melanoma cells transformation from non-malignant to invasive ones is accompanied by the loss of E-cadherin and overexpression of N-cadherin. It has been suggested, however, that not N-cadherin itself had been responsible for the start of melanoma cells dissemination and metastasis formation [63]. Observations have revealed that the deregulation of E- and N-cadherin expression is involved in tumourigenesis and cancer progression also in other skin cancers—MCC, SCC and BCC [52, 58, 64, 65].

2.3.1. E-cadherin

The important role of E-cadherin expression for the malignant transformation of melanoma cells and SCC has been confirmed in numerous tissue samples assembled in tissue microarrays of human malignant melanoma and SCC as well as in selected cell lines, including A375, SK-MEL-24, MV3 and M14 melanoma cell lines. As a conclusion of this analysis, Tang et al. [66] have postulated the reverse correlation between the E-cadherin expression level and the expression of ubiquitin protein ligase E3C (UBE3C), which positively regulates tumour growth and metastasis by inducing the mesenchymal phenotype of melanoma cells. In melanoma, E-cadherin expression has been also shown to be correlated with the altered expression of microRNA (miRNA). Analysis of frozen melanoma tissue section demonstrated that the decreased expression of mi-R200a, mi-R200c, and miR-203, previously described as contributors of melanoma metastasis, correlated with down-regulation of E-cadherin and growing tumour thickness. These data reveal miRNA role in the regulation of E-cadherin expression in the course of melanoma progression [67].

α-catulin is a cytoplasmic molecule, overexpressed in melanoma that has been recognized as a negative regulator of E-cadherin expression, consequently promoting melanoma progression. It has been confirmed in α-catulin knockdown experiments, where the enhanced melanoma cells binding to keratinocytes as well as up-regulated E-cadherin expression have been observed resulting in the lower migratory and invasive potential of melanoma cells [68].

In BCC, it has been observed that tumour progression is accompanied by the decreased membranous expression of E-cadherin. Additionally, the increased nuclear localization of E-cadherin, as well as nuclear translocation of β-catenin, has been shown [52].

Analysis of 227 tissue sections of MCC has revealed weak and mainly cytoplasmic staining for E-cadherin and there were no statistically significant differences in the immunoreactivity between various tumour locations (primary, local or distant metastasis), suggesting that E-cadherin is not relevant for MCC progression [69].

The loss of E-cadherin has been suggested to be a trigger of cancer progression especially because of the reduced cell-cell adhesion and possible stimulation of T cell factor (TCF)-regulated genes, responsible for proliferation and invasion (c-myc, cyclin D1, fibronectin and matrilysin), as an effect of released β-catenin migration to nucleus [19]. The expression of E-cadherin is regulated by different transcription factors including grainyhead-like 3 (Grl-3) factor, which has been shown to participate in the regulation of differentiation and migration of epithelial cells during embryonic development. In normal human keratinocytes (HaCat) and human SCC (A431) cells, the reverse correlation between Grl-3 and E-cadherin expression level has been shown and the induced overexpression of Grl-3 in A431 cells has led to the increased motility and invasion of cancer cells as an effect of E-cadherin down-regulation [65].

Another transcription factor, regulating E-cadherin expression, is Slug. Its presence has been confirmed in multiple melanoma tissue sections, and higher expression has been attributed to nevi than to primary or metastatic melanoma. Such observations have suggested that higher Slug expression is required at the beginning of melanocyte neoplastic transformation but not during melanoma progression. However, in melanocytes and melanoma cells cultured *in vitro*, the exogenous expression of Slug has resulted in the down-regulated expression of E-cadherin and up-regulated expression of N-cadherin and subsequently more efficient cellular migration and invasion [70].

E-cadherin regulatory potential has been attributed also to NOTCH receptors and their signalling pathways. In a set of tissue samples from skin cancer and their adjacent normal skin, the analysis of NOTCH expression has shown the up-regulated receptor expression along with increased Snail and decreased E-cadherin expression in cancer tissue. Simultaneously, the up-regulation/inhibition of NOTCH signalling in A341 cells has resulted in changes in E-cadherin expression, decrease or increase, respectively. The observed effects of NOTCH alteration in SCC have been mediated by Snail up-regulation and subsequent E-cadherin promoter methylation [71].

The experiments with induced E-cadherin suppression in Ras-transformed keratinocytes have revealed the importance of E-cadherin role in SCC neoplastic transformation. E-cadherin absence has increased Src activity leading to the up-regulated expression of FAK that supported the progression of tumour malignancy also by the following deregulation of E-cadherin-dependent adhesion [72].

In melanoma, cadherin switch has been widely described but its molecular mechanism is still not fully explained. To deal with this, Hao et al. [73] using a set of melanoma cell lines from different stages of progression have analysed the expression profile of E- and N-cadherin, PI3K/PTEN pathway components and Snail, Slug and Twist transcription factors. They have shown the correlation between the loss of PTEN activity and E- to N-cadherin switch. The observed cadherin changes have been regulated at the transcriptional level by Twist and Snail, which activity in PTEN-null cells was stimulated by constitutively active PI3K. It has also been reported that the membranous localization of E-cadherin is not controlled by PI3K/PTEN but more likely depends on cadherin-β-catenin interaction [73]. The study on a vast range of primary melanoma tissue samples has confirmed the correlation between down-regulated PTEN expression and 'cadherin switch'. Additionally, this study has shown the linkage of these markers with melanoma progression parameter, that is, Breslow thickness of primary tumours, ulceration and tumour stage. The immunohistochemical detection of E- and N-cadherin as well as PTEN has been conducted and the statistical analysis of results has shown that E-cadherin, unlike N-cadherin, possesses a predictor value. Low E-cadherin expression level has been correlated with a better survival prognosis, without relapses and distant metastasis [74].

Cadherin-mediated adhesion is regarded as a dynamic process adapting to the epithelial tissue remodelling during development and wound healing but also during carcinogenesis. Considering this fact, the proteolytic cleavage of E-cadherin has been suggested as a mechanism of rapid adhesion changes. The role in E-cadherin shedding has been attributed to different ADAMs (a disintegrin-like and metalloproteinase) and MMPs (matrix metalloproteinases) [75]. As a result of its action, a decreased membranous E-cadherin expression and an increased level of 80-kDa soluble E-cadherin fragment (sE-cadherin) in tumour microenvironment have been reported in human SCC clinical tissue samples and SCC mouse model. Moreover, sE-cadherin binding with HER/IGF-1R has been observed, and the consequent initiation of pro-oncogenic signalling, resulting in cancer cell migration, proliferation and invasion, has been reported. Thus, the sE-cadherin has been suggested as a potential therapeutic target in skin cancer treatment [76]. The potential therapeutic value of anti-sE-cadherin antibody has been suggested in SCC model PAM212 cell line. This antibody has inhibited tumour growth, enhanced cell death and silenced the pro-survival pathways by the inhibition of proto-oncogenes (RTKs, IAPs and MDM2) and stimulation of tumour suppressor genes (PTEN and p53) [77].

The diagnostic usefulness of E-cadherin expression changes has been determined for melanoma versus Spitz tumours distinction (Spitz tumour; a benign cutaneous melanocytic tumour). Such distinction is often problematic because of poor reproducibility of Spitz tumour features and therefore unequivocally delineated diagnostic criteria. The obtained results have suggested that the quantitative differences rather than qualitative irregularities in E-cadherin immunoreactivity could have diagnostic potential [78].

Studies in a variety of melanoma cell lines have shown that the restoration of E-cadherin expression leads to the renewing of communication with keratinocytes and inhibition of melanoma cells invasion [79]. E-cadherin-restored expression has also been observed in SCC cells treated with flavonoids. Highly invasive A431-III cells selected from the parental A341 cell line have been analysed. The invasive potential of A341-III cells has been attributed to their mesenchymal-like phenotype resulting from 'cadherin switch'. Cells have been treated with plant flavonoids: luteolin and quercetin. They are known for their anticancer activity resulting in the inhibition of cell growth, induction of apoptosis and differentiation, as well as the diminution of tumour angiogenesis, cancer cells adhesion, invasion and metastasis. As an effect, A341-III cells have remodelled their morphology to more epithelial-like. It was accompanied by changes in the EMT markers expression level, including down-regulation of N-cadherin and up-regulation of E-cadherin, leading to the renovation of the cell-cell junctions. Therefore, both flavonoids used have been suggested to have chemopreventive, anticancerogenic or chemotherapeutic activity, mainly through their EMT-reverting potential [80].

2.3.2. P-cadherin

The role of P-cadherin in carcinogenesis is ambiguous. It has been shown to promote the invasive behaviour of cancer cells; however, in melanoma it has been reported as a tumour growth suppressor [81]. Clinical data have shown that in general, melanocytic cells in compound nevi and melanomas express E- and P-cadherins; however, a reduction in the expression thereof has been observed in correlation to the depth of melanoma cells dermal localization. It has been suggested that this loss represents melanoma cells' adaptation to the changed microenvironment of the dermis and makes them less dependent on microenvironmental stimulation leading to the increased cell proliferation and melanoma progression [82]. Additionally, the potential usefulness of P-cadherin as a prognostic marker for immunohistochemical detection and diagnosis in patients with primary melanoma of less than 2-mm tumour thickness has been suggested [83]. In melanoma, the alteration of P-cadherin expression in a tissue section of different stages has been shown together with its switch from membranous to cytoplasmic localization. These changes have strongly correlated with patient's survival prognosis, suggesting P-cadherin as a useful marker of melanoma progression [84].

2.3.3. N-cadherin

The analysis of E-, N- and P-cadherin expression has been conducted in human MCCs and in Merkel cells of the healthy epidermis. It has shown the high level of N-cadherin expression in all MCCs with a simultaneous lack of immunoreactivity in the healthy epidermis. The strong E- and P-cadherin positive reaction of Merkel cells and only partial positive immunoreaction for both cadherins in MCCs have also been shown. These results have suggested that 'cadherin switch' takes place also during Merkel cells neoplastic transformation. Additionally, the loss of P-cadherin expression in MCCs has been linked with a more advanced clinical stages, while its expression has been significantly more frequent in primary MCC [64]. The study of Vlahova and co-workers has shown the similarity in P-cadherin immunoreactivity between primary tumours and distance metastasis of MCCs, while the lymph node metastases have exhibited a lower level of P-cadherin expression. Additionally, the analysis suggested that the membranous expression of P-cadherin in MCCs positively correlates with a prolonged survival prognosis [85]. Depending on the expressed cadherin type, melanoma cells, compared to melanocytes, have been shown to possess different preferences in cell-cell communication. Melanocytes interact mostly with their neighbouring keratinocytes, while melanoma cells preferentially form their gap junction with fibroblasts and among themselves. It has also been observed that gap junction could be established between melanoma cells and N-cadherin expressing endothelial cells, suggesting that the gap junction formation is rather dependent on N-cadherin expression than cell-type-specific [79]. N-cadherin-dependent heterotypic cell-cell adhesion has been described between fibroblasts and WM1205Lu melanoma cells with Smad7 overexpression. In this model, cells have been arrested in their invasion abilities. It has been suggested that the subsequent loss of N-cadherin expression during the following steps of melanoma progression may be a key factor for metastasis formation, because melanoma cells by losing their interaction with fibroblasts become able to migrate to distant metastatic sites, and after that N-cadherin expression can be restored [86]. Additionally, the role of N-cadherin expression for primary (WM793, WM115) and malignant melanoma cells (WM1205Lu, WM266-4 cell lines) proliferation has been analysed with the use of specific N-cadherin siRNA. The observed decrease in N-cadherin expression level up-regulates the cell cycle inhibitors p15, p16, p21 and p27 expression leading to cell cycle arrest in G1 phase and significantly down-regulates AKT, ERK and β-catenin signalling, resulting in the inhibition of cell proliferation [87].

2.3.4. T-cadherin

During malignant transformation of melanocytes, the expression of T-cadherin on both mRNA and protein levels decreases, mainly due to the repression of CDH13 promoter activity by BRN2 transcription factor [36], and finally disappears in human malignant melanomas [88]. Down-regulation of T-cadherin expression is accompanied by a higher growth, proliferation, migration and invasion of malignant cells *in vitro*. Re-expression of T-cadherin in human melanoma cells, via stable transfection, draws back these effects *in vitro* and in a xenograft mouse model *in vivo* [89]. Re-expression of T-cadherin also elevates the apoptotic rate of melanoma cells *in vitro* through down-regulation of AKT and FoxO3a, which is in turn accompanied by the down-regulation of anti-apoptotic molecules BCL-2, BCL-x and clustering from one site and deactivation of transcription factors CREB and AP-1 from another site [90]. Furthermore, ectopic up-regulated T-cadherin sensitizes the apoptosis induced by treatment with CD95/Fas antibody CH-11 [90]. Contradictory results have been demonstrated for a fully mouse model of melanoma, where up-regulated T-cadherin acted oppositely at the same time: as a positive and a negative regulator of mouse melanoma development [91]. Namely, it has been shown that the overexpression of T-cadherin in B16F10 mouse melanoma promotes primary tumour growth due to the recruitment of mesenchymal stromal cells, as well as enhances cell motility, invasiveness and metastasis formation in BDF1 mice in parallel with the inhibition of neovascularization of primary melanoma sites [91]. This apparent discrepancy has been explained by the recent study, which showed that in the species-specific environment T-cadherin-overexpressed melanoma cells up-regulated the level of pro-oncogenic integrins, chemokines, adhesion molecules and extracellular matrix components, which in turn increased the invasive potential of tumour cells [92]. It is believed that T-cadherin is an endogenous suppressor of keratinocyte proliferation by delaying the G2/M phase progression [93]. It has been shown that T-cadherin is also a suppressor of keratinocyte migration and invasion, and the inactivation of T-cadherin, through allelic loss or hypermethylation of a gene-promoter region, may induce keratinocyte-derived aggressive epithelial tumours with high metastatic potential [94]. Inverse correlations between T-cadherin expression and pre-cancerous (AK, BD), benign (KA) and malignant skin diseases (invasive SCC and BCC) have been well documented in immunohistochemical and *in vitro* studies [88, 95–98]. In other works, the expression of T-cadherin was found to be higher in superficial, nodular or infiltrative BCCs [99] as well as in differentiated/primary SCCs [100] than in normal keratinocytes; however, it was mainly restricted to the leading fronts of the tumours, where the up-regulated T-cadherin induced a morphological spread and inhibited cell invasive potential [100]. It has been shown that ectopic up-regulation of T-cadherin increased SCC cell-matrix adhesiveness by promoting the retention of both β1 integrin and epidermal growth factor receptor (EGFR) in lipid raft domains, and by increasing integrin β1-activation in parallel with the suppression of tyrosine phosphorylation of EGFR [101, 102].

The molecular mechanisms underlying T-cadherin function as a guardian maintaining a non-invasive phenotype of keratinocytes are different from those typically associated with EMT and consist in the indirect negative regulation of EGFR pathway activity; gain or loss of T-cadherin expression switches EGFR signalling off or on, respectively. On the other hand, loss of T-cadherin in SCC may lead to ligand-dependent EGFR hyperactivation and acquiring invasive and aggressive phenotype [102]. It has been shown that co-culture of SCC cells with epithelial cells stimulated ECs to produce EGF [103], which in turn facilitated transendothelial migration of T-cadherin-silenced cells, and their growth within the invaded stroma [104]. In human A431 cells (SCC), EGF-induced phosphorylation of EGFR and resulting downstream signalling through p38MAPK, Erk1/2 and Rac1 contributed to the re-localization of T-cadherin within the plasma membrane from dispersed to focused in intercellular junctions, where it indirectly co-localizes with activated EGFR. Being in complex with p-EGFR, T-cadherin acts as an attenuator for EGFR signalling and its loss shifts the balance between Erk1/2-p38MAPK in favour of Erk1/2 activity [104]. In this way, plasma membrane-associated T-cadherin functions as a regulatory factor, which promotes or represses EGF effects mediated by MAP kinases.

2.3.5. Proteins interacting with cadherins

Cadherins as adhesion receptors are players in the interdependent adhesion network and it is still an issue to decipher the mechanism of their direct interaction with other adhesion proteins. Studies show that E- and N-cadherins participate in the adhesion along with integrins and their interaction with $\alpha_2\beta_1$-integrin has been examined in melanoma cell line and tissue microarray and tissue section. Simultaneous expression of E- and N-cadherins with $\alpha_2\beta_1$-integrin has been reported in numerous primary and metastatic melanoma cells, and the differentiated localization of such complexes has been observed suggesting their independency. It has also been suggested that $\alpha_2\beta_1$-integrin/N-cadherin complex interplays in the regulation of melanoma cells invasion and migration, while the $\alpha_2\beta_1$-integrin/E-cadherin complex affects cell-cell adhesion [105].

Another receptor cross-talking with E-cadherin is EGFR, which overexpression has been commonly reported in many types of cancer, including skin cancer, and this interaction is of particular interest regarding tumour progression. The association between both receptors is realized via domain of β-catenin, which has been shown to participate in ligand-induced E-cadherin signalling resulting in the inhibition of EGF-dependent cell growth. It has been suggested that homophilic binding of E-cadherin interrupts the activation-signalling pathway subsequent to EGFR without blocking receptor activation [106]. On the other hand, activated EGFR has been described as an upstream regulator of Twist expression leading to its overexpression and alternating E-cadherin down-regulation together with EMT of SCC cells. These observations have suggested mutual regulation between E-cadherin and EGFR [107]. Additionally, the analysis of head and neck SCC has revealed that E-cadherin loss is accompanied by the transcriptional up-regulation of EGFR and results in the increased cell proliferation due to enhanced EGFR signalling [108]. EGFR has also been reported to regulate E-cadherin-dependent cell-cell adhesion by the modulation of E-cadherin assembly with actin cytoskeleton and vinculin, and EGFR activation has led to the distraction of cadherin-vinculin-actin complexes [109].

Interesting interaction has also been described between E-cadherin and caveolin-1, which is generally recognized as a tumour suppressor; however, its contribution to metastasis formation has also been described. In melanoma cells, the co-expression and observed co-localization of E-cadherin and caveolin-1 have resulted in the decreased cell proliferation, enhanced cell death and reduced subcutaneous tumour growth. Despite the reduced E-cadherin expression, related with 'cadherin switch' occurring in melanoma progression, caveolin-1 expression has increased in the analysed metastatic melanomas and correlated with higher tumour malignancy. Due to collectively observed N-cadherin expression, their potential cooperation with caveolin-1 in lung metastasis formation has been suggested [110].

3. Alterations in glycophenotype of cells in skin cancers

Nowadays, instead of the conventional histopathological diagnosis, the antibody or lectin histochemistry approaches are used to distinguish between normal, pre-neoplastic, benign and malignant skin tissues and to improve a quantitative assessment of cancer progression [111]. For example, AK, KA, SCC and BCC show lower expression of high mannose-type and/or hybrid-type N-glycans as well as fucose α1,2-linked to galactose residue (H antigen) compared to normal tissue. However, cutaneous tumours (SCC, BCC, invasive melanoma) display higher expression of truncated mucin-type O-glycan, that is, T antigen (Galβ1-3Gal-

NAc residue) than normal tissue [111–113]. Mannose-type and/or hybrid-type N-glycans and T antigen can be used as markers for the distinction between BCC and TE [111]. Higher-expression levels of β-galactoside α-2,3 sialyltransferase (ST3Gal I) and higher cell-surface reactivity with *Maackia amurensis* agglutinin (MAA), which recognizes sialic acid α2,3-linked to Gal residue, allow to distinguish AK and SCC from KA, BCC and normal epidermis [113, 114]. MCCs do not show expression of neither α2,3-linked sialic acid nor H antigen [115]. By contrast, the expression of β-galactoside α-2,6-sialyltransferase (ST6Gal I) is higher in skin tumours with a greater potential for invasion and metastasis, as in the case of SCC, BCC and melanoma [114, 116]. The difference in the expression level of α2,6-linked sialic acid distinguishes premalignant AK stage from the invasive SCC stage of skin cancer. Unlike the normal and non-malignant epidermis, pre-malignant biopsies and malignant cells from patients with BCC and SCC are positive with the sialylated Le^a structure [117]. Additional O-acetylation at C-9 of sialic acid residue is prominent in melanoma and BCC [116]. It has been shown that very intense binding of mistletoe lectin I (ML-I; which is specific for galactose and Neu5Acα2-6Galβ-) and of *Helix pomatia* agglutinin (HPA; it selectively binds to T and Tn antigens) was positively correlated with the metastasis of melanoma and were not expressed in benign nevus cells, and thus they are predictors of poor prognosis [118–120].

4. Glycosylation of cadherins the skin cancers

Cadherins, like other adhesion proteins, are strongly glycosylated, as they possessed a number of potential N-glycosylation sites in their extracellular domain and O-glycosylation sites in the cytoplasmic domain. Based on the analysis of amino acid sequence, human E-cadherin possesses four potential N-glycosylation sites in its extracellular domain, located at Asn residues 554, 566, 618 and 633 [28], in EC4 and EC5 [121]. N-cadherin ectodomain has been reported to contain eight potential N-glycosylation sites, but only three of them, located in EC2 and EC3, were effectively N-glycosylated [122].

Despite the described redundancy of possible N-glycosylation sites, it has been shown that up to 20% of total molecular mass of cadherin may come from the N-glycan component, and it is the most prominent cadherin post-translational modification. In a culture, more abundant N-glycosylation of E-cadherin has been observed in sparsely growing cells than in dense ones. E-cadherin from sparse cultures has been shown to possess mainly complex-type and lack the high mannose-type N-glycans. On the contrary, N-glycans of E-cadherin from cells growing in a dense culture have composed mainly of high mannose-type and only small amounts of complex-type N-glycans have been detected. Furthermore, the differences in E-cadherin turnover have been reported in respect to its glycosylation status. In general, the level of E-cadherin expression in a dense culture is lowered. Also, the constitution and stability of AJs have been affected by E-cadherin changed N-glycans structure and quantity. The high level of E-cadherin N-glycosylation in a sparse culture has led to unstable adhesion and it has been correlated with cell proliferation. On the other hand, in a dense culture, E-cadherin decoration with high mannose-type N-glycans has resulted in the formation of stable AJs and stronger adhesion [10].

Aberrations in N-oligosaccharides composition are also commonly attributed to cancer transformation and progression in various types of cancer cells [123]. The biantennary complex-type and high mannose-type oligosaccharides are characteristic for normal cells, while progressive malignant transformation of cancer cells is accompanied by the synthesis of more branched (tri-, tetra- or even pentaantennary) N-glycans of complex-types, elongated with poly-N-acetyllactosamine chains [124].

There are also some data concerning the abundance and diverse structural composition of N-glycans attached to cadherin observed mostly in melanoma among other skin cancers [125–128] and N-glycosylation role in cadherin function has been confirmed [29]. O-glycosylation of cadherins has also been described, and especially concerning E-cadherin, their role in the inhibition of protein trafficking has been suggested [129].

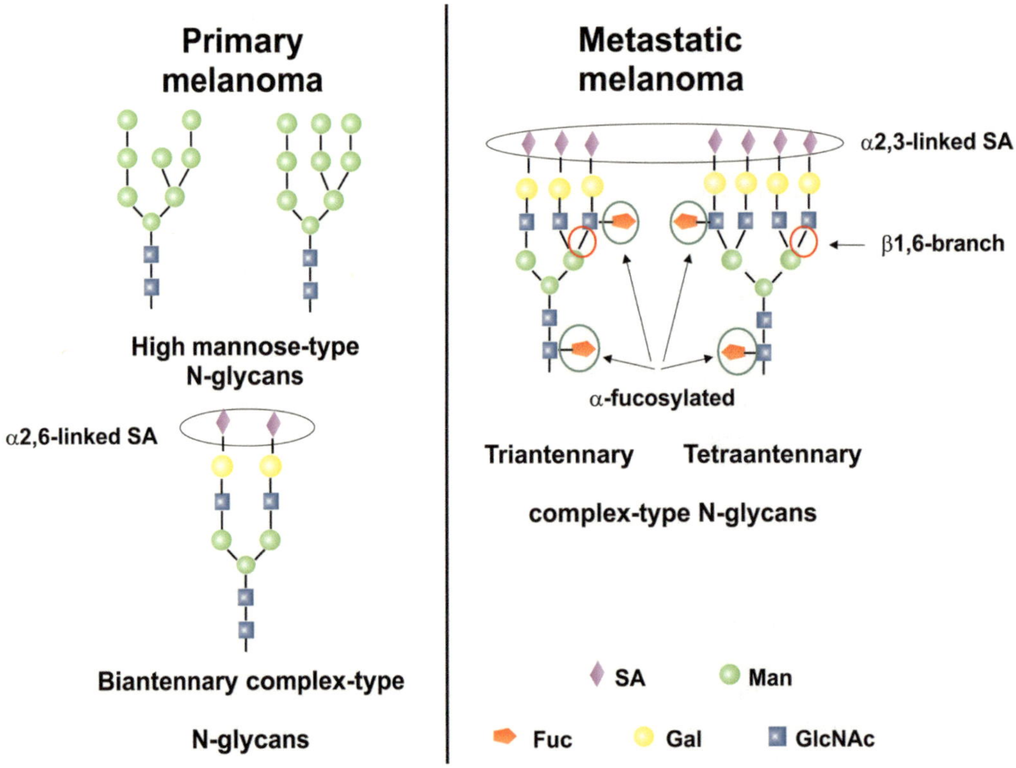

Figure 1. N-glycan structures detected on N-cadherin in melanoma. Gal, galactose; GlcNAc, N-acetylglucosamine; Fuc, fucose; Man, mannose; and SA, sialic acids.

The changed N-glycosylation of cadherins (E- and N-cadherin) has been described in melanoma cells of various cell lines [126–128, 130]. However, this problem has not been studied as extensively as in other types of cancer. The detailed N-glycans analysis showed that N-cadherin from primary melanoma cells possesses mainly high mannose-type and biantennary complex-type oligosaccharides with α2,6-linked sialic acids, while N-cadherin from metastatic cells possesses mostly tri- and tetraantennary complex-type oligosaccharides, with β1,6-branches, highly α-fucosylated and with α2,3-linked sialic acids (**Figure 1**) [126, 128, 130]. Such observations are in line with observations that more branched N-glycans, especially β1,6-branched oligosaccharides, are associated with a higher motility of tumour cells and its more invasive behaviour. In mouse melanoma model B16F10 cells, E-cadherin was shown to be a target protein for N-acetylglucosaminyltransferase III (GnT-III) action, which is suggested to be a suppressor of the invasive phenotype. In GnT-III-transfected melanoma cells, E-cadherin has been found to bear the bisecting GlcNAc structures which prolonged E-cadherin turnover and resistance to proteolysis. As an effect, the enhancement of cadherin-dependent cellular adhesion leading to the suppression of metastasis has been observed [125].

5. Conclusions

It is commonly accepted that cadherins play a crucial role in cancer progression. Their expression abnormality taking place in different stages of skin cancer progression as well as changes in their glycosylation status leading to adhesion impairment precedes tumour cells dissemination and metastasis formation. The detailed analysis of cadherin-related glycosylation changes in cancer cells could be a key for better understanding of the nature of malignant transformation process and may open new opportunities for the development of more effective anticancer therapeutics and diagnostic tools.

Acknowledgements

Writing of this manuscript was supported in part by grants from the Institute of Zoology, Jagiellonian University in Krakow (K/ZDS/005403) and from the National Science Centre, Poland (2013/11/B/NZ4/04315).

Author details

Marcelina E. Janik*, Dorota Hoja-Łukowicz and Małgorzata Przybyło

*Address all correspondence to: marcelina.janik@uj.edu.pl

Department of Glycoconjugate Biochemistry, Institute of Zoology, Jagiellonian University, Kraków, Poland

References

[1] Bassagañas S, Carvalho S, Dias AM, Pérez-Garay M, Ortiz MR, Figueras J, Reis CA, Pinho SS, Peracaula R. Pancreatic cancer cell glycosylation regulates cell adhesion and invasion through the modulation of $\alpha2\beta1$ integrin and E-cadherin function. PLoS One. 2014;9(5):e98595. doi: 10.1371/journal.pone.0098595

[2] Angst BD, Marcozzi C, Magee AI. The cadherin superfamily: diversity in form and function. J Cell Sci. 2001;114(4):629–641.

[3] Dames SA, Bang E, Haüssinger D, Ahrens T, Engel J, Grzesiek S. Insights into the low adhesive capacity of human T-cadherin from the NMR structure of its N-terminal extracellular domain. J Biol Chem. 2008; 283(34):23485–23495.

[4] van Roy F, Berx G. The cell-cell adhesion molecule E-cadherin. Cell Mol Life Sci. 2008;65:3756–3788.

[5] Brooke MA, Nitoiu D, Kelsell DP. Cell–cell connectivity: desmosomes and disease. J Pathol. 2012;226:158–171.

[6] Chen Y-H, Stewart DB, Nelson WJ. Coupling assembly of the E-cadherin/b-catenin complex to efficient endoplasmic reticulum exit and basal–lateral membrane targeting of E-cadherin in polarized MDCK cells. J Cell Biol. 1999;144:687–699.

[7] Niessen CM, Gottardi CJ. Molecular components of the adherens junction. Biochim Biophys Acta. 2008;1778(3):562–571.

[8] Davis MA, Ireton RC, Reynolds AB. A core function for p120-catenin in cadherin turnover. J Cell Biol. 2003;163(3):525–534.

[9] Herzig M, Savarese F, Novatchkova M, Semb H, Christofori G. Tumor progression induced by the loss of E-cadherin in dependent on beta-catenin/Tcf-mediated Wnt signaling. Oncogene. 2007;26(16):2290–2298.

[10] Liwosz A, Lei T, Kukuruzinska MA. N-Glycosylation affects the molecular organization and stability of E-cadherin junctions. J Biol Chem. 2006;281(32): 23138–23149.

[11] Shapiro L, Weis WI. Structure and biochemistry of cadherins and catenins. Cold Spring Harb Perspect Biol. 2009;1(3):a003053. doi: 10.1101/cshperspect.a003053.

[12] Green KJ, Getsios S, Troyanovsky S, Godsel LM. Intercellular junction assembly, dynamics, and homeostasis. Cold Spring Harb Perspect Biol. 2010;2(2):a000125. doi: 10.1101/cshperspect.a000125.

[13] Canel M, Serrels A, Frame MC, Brunton VG. E-cadherin-integrin crosstalk in cancer invasion and metastasis. J Cell Sci. 2013;126(2):393–401. doi: 10.1242/jcs.100115.

[14] Jeanes A, Gottardi CJ, Yap AS. Cadherins and cancer: how does cadherin dysfunction promote tumor progression? Oncogene. 2008;27(55):6920–6929. doi: 10.1038/onc.2008.343.

[15] Gallin WJ, Edelman GM, Cunningham BA. Characterization of L-CAM, a major cell adhesion molecule from embryonic liver cells. Proc Natl Acad Sci USA. 1983;80(4):1038–1042.

[16] Ogou SI, Yoshida-Noro C, Takeichi M. Calcium-dependent cell-cell adhesion molecules common to hepatocytes and teratocarcinoma stem cells. J Cell Biol. 1983;97(3):944–948.

[17] Peyriéras N, Hyafil F, Louvard D, Ploegh HL, Jacob F. Uvomorulin: a nonintegral membrane protein of early mouse embryo. Proc Natl Acad Sci USA. 1983;80(20):6274–6277.

[18] Halbleib JM, Nelson WJ. Cadherins in development: cell adhesion, sorting, and tissue morphogenesis. Genes Dev. 2006;20(23):3199–3214.

[19] Hazan RB, Qiao R, Keren RT, Badano I, Suyama K. Cadherin switch in tumor progression. Ann NY Acad Sci. 2004;1014:155–163. doi: 10.1196/annals.1294.016

[20] Inuzuka H, Redies C, Takeichi M. Differential expression of R- and N-cadherin in neural and mesodermal tissues during early chicken development. Development. 1991;113(3):959–967.

[21] Vestweber D, Winderlich M, Cagna G, Nottebaum AF. Cell adhesion dynamics at endothelial junctions: VE-cadherin as a major player. Trends Cell Biol. 2009;19(1):8–15. doi: 10.1016/j.tcb.2008.10.001.

[22] Prakash S, Swaminathan U. β catenin in health: a review. J Oral Maxillofac Pathol. 2015;19(2):230–238. doi: 10.4103/0973-029X.164537.

[23] van Roy F. Beyond E-cadherin: roles of other cadherin superfamily members in cancer. Nat Rev Cancer. 2014;14(2):121–134. doi: 10.1038/nrc3647.

[24] Samuelov L, Sprecher E, Paus R. The role of P-cadherin in skin biology and skin pathology: lessons from the hair follicle. Cell Tissue Res. 2015;360(3):761–771. doi: 10.1007/s00441-015-2114-y.

[25] Shan WS, Tanaka H, Phillips GR, Arndt K, Yoshida M, Colman DR, Shapiro L. Functional cis-heterodimers of N- and R-cadherins. J Cell Biol. 2000;148(3):579–590.

[26] Zhu B, Chappuis-Flament S, Wong E, Jensen IE, Gumbiner BM, Leckband D. Functional analysis of the structural basis of homophilic cadherin adhesion. Biophys J. 2003;84(6):4033–4042.

[27] Stemmler MP. Cadherins in development and cancer. Mol Biosyst. 2008;4(8):835–850. doi: 10.1039/b719215k.

[28] Zhao H, Sun L, Wang L, Xu Z, Zhou F, Su J, Jin J, Yang Y, Hu Y, Zha X. N-glycosylation at Asn residues 554 and 566 of E-cadherin affects cell cycle progression through

extracellular signal-regulated protein kinase signaling pathway. Acta Biochim Biophys Sin (Shanghai). 2008;40(2):140–148.

[29] Pinho SS, Seruca R, Gärtner F, Yamaguchi Y, Gu J, Taniguchi N, Reis CA. Modulation of E-cadherin function and dysfunction by N-glycosylation. Cell Mol Life Sci. 2011;68(6):1011–1020. doi: 10.1007/s00018-010-0595-0.

[30] Nose A, Takeichi M. A novel cadherin adhesion molecule: Its expression pattern associated with implantation and organogenesis of mouse embryos. J Cell Biol. 1986; 103:2649–2658.

[31] Li L, Fukunaga-Kalabis M, Yu H, Xu X, Kong J, Lee JT, Herlyn M. Human dermal stem cells differentiate into functional epidermal melanocytes. J Cell Sci. 2010;123(Pt 6):853–860. doi: 10.1242/jcs.061598.

[32] Keswell D, Kidson SH, Davids LM. Melanocyte migration is influenced by E-cadherin-dependent adhesion of keratinocytes in both two- and three-dimensional in vitro wound models. Cell Biol Int. 2015;39(2):169–176. doi: 10.1002/cbin.10350.

[33] Perlis C, Herlyn M. Recent advances in melanoma biology. Oncologist. 2004;9(2):182–187.

[34] Jouneau A, Yu YQ, Pasdar M, Larue L. Plasticity of cadherin-catenin expression in the melanocyte lineage. Pigment Cell Res. 2000;13(4):260–272.

[35] Derycke LD, Bracke ME. N-cadherin in the spotlight of cell-cell adhesion, differentiation, embryogenesis, invasion and signalling. Int J Dev Biol. 2004;48(5-6):463–476.

[36] Ellmann L, Joshi MB, Resink TJ, Bosserhoff AK, Kuphal S. BRN2 is a transcriptional repressor of CDH13 (T-cadherin) in melanoma cells. Lab Invest. 2012; 92:1788–1800.

[37] Cavallaro U, Schaffhauser B, Christofori G. Cadherins and the tumour progression: is it all in a switch? Cancer Lett. 2002;176(2):123–128.

[38] Paluncic J, Kovacevic Z, Jansson PJ, Kalinowski D, Merlot AM, Huang ML, Lok HC, Sahni S, Lane DJ, Richardson DR. Roads to melanoma: key pathways and emerging players in melanoma progression and oncogenic signaling. Biochim Biophys Acta. 2016;1863(4):770–784. doi: 10.1016/j.bbamcr.2016.01.025.

[39] Lupia A, Peppicelli S, Witort E, Bianchini F, Carloni V, Pimpinelli N, Urso C, Borgognoni L, Capaccioli S, Calorini L, Lulli M. CD63 tetraspanin is a negative driver of epithelial-to-mesenchymal transition in human melanoma cells. J Invest Dermatol. 2014;134(12): 2947–2956. doi: 10.1038/jid.2014.258.

[40] Yang J, Weinberg RA. Epithelial-mesenchymal transition: at the crossroads of development and tumor metastasis. Dev Cell. 2008;14(6):818–829. doi: 10.1016/j.devcel.2008.05.009.

[41] Verrill C, Cerundolo L, Mckee C, White M, Kartsonaki C, Fryer E, Morris E, Brewster S, Ratnayaka I, Marsden L, Lilja H, Muschel R, Lu X, Hamdy F, Bryant RJ. Altered

expression of epithelial-to-mesenchymal transition proteins in extraprostatic prostate cancer. Oncotarget. 2016;7(2):1107–1119. doi: 10.18632/oncotarget.6689.

[42] Thiery JP, Acloque H, Huang RY, Nieto MA. Epithelial-mesenchymal transitions in development and disease. Cell. 2009;139(5):871–890. doi: 10.1016/j.cell.2009.11.007.

[43] Honjo M, Tanihara H, Suzuki S, Tanaka T, Honda Y, Takeichi M. Differential expression of cadherin adhesion receptors in neural retina of the postnatal mouse. Invest Ophthalmol Vis Sci. 2000;41(2):546–551.

[44] Carver EA, Jiang R, Lan Y, Oram KF, Gridley T. The mouse snail gene encodes a key regulator of the epithelial-mesenchymal transition. Mol Cell Biol. 2001;21(23):8184–8188.

[45] Xu L, Overbeek PA, Reneker LW. Systematic analysis of E-, N- and P-cadherin expression in mouse eye development. Exp Eye Res. 2002;74(6):753–760.

[46] Barrette K, Van Kelst S, Wouters J, Marasigan V, Fieuws S, Agostinis P, van den Oord J, Garmyn M. Epithelial-mesenchymal transition during invasion of cutaneous squamous cell carcinoma is paralleled by AKT activation. Br J Dermatol. 2014;171(5):1014–1021. doi: 10.1111/bjd.12967.

[47] von Maltzan K, Li Y, Rundhaug JE, Hudson LG, Fischer SM, Kusewitt DF. Role of the Slug transcription factor in chemically-induced skin cancer. J Clin Med. 2006;5(2):21. doi: 10.3390/jcm5020021.

[48] Majima Y, Hirakawa S, Kito Y, Suzuki H, Koide M, Fukamizu H, Tokura Y. Twist1 as a possible biomarker for metastatic basal cell carcinoma. Acta Derm Venereol. 2012;92(6): 621–622. doi: 10.2340/00015555-1422.

[49] Toll A, Masferrer E, Hernández-Ruiz ME, Ferrandiz-Pulido C, Yébenes M, Jaka A, Tuneu A, Jucglà A, Gimeno J, Baró T, Casado B, Gandarillas A, Costa I, Mojal S, Peña R, de Herreros AG, García-Patos V, Pujol RM, Hernández-Muñoz I. Epithelial to mesenchymal transition markers are associated with an increased metastatic risk in primary cutaneous squamous cell carcinomas but are attenuated in lymph node metastases. J Dermatol Sci. 2013;72(2):93–102. doi: 10.1016/j.jdermsci.2013.07.001.

[50] Lan YJ, Chen H, Chen JQ, Lei QH, Zheng M, Shao ZR. Immunolocalization of vimentin, keratin 17, Ki-67, involucrin, β-catenin and E-cadherin in cutaneous squamous cell carcinoma. Pathol Oncol Res. 2014;20(2):263–266. doi: 10.1007/s12253-013-9690-5.

[51] Geng S, Guo Y, Wang Q, Li L, Wang J. Cancer stem-like cells enriched with CD29 and CD44 markers exhibit molecular characteristics with epithelial-mesenchymal transition in squamous cell carcinoma. Arch Dermatol Res. 2013;305(1):35–47. doi: 10.1007/s00403-012-1260-2.

[52] Papanikolaou S, Bravou V, Gyftopoulos K, Nakas D, Repanti M, Papadaki H. ILK expression in human basal cell carcinoma correlates with epithelial-mesenchymal

transition markers and tumour invasion. Histopathology. 2010;56(6):799–809. doi: 10.1111/j.1365-2559.2010.03556.x.

[53] Chen LL, Jaimes N, Barker CA, Busam KJ, Marghoob AA. Desmoplastic melanoma: a review. J Am Acad Dermatol. 2013;68(5):825–833. doi: 10.1016/j.jaad.2012.10.041.

[54] Garrido MC, Requena L, Kutzner H, Ortiz P, Pérez-Gómez B, Rodriguez-Peralto JL. Desmoplastic melanoma: expression of epithelial-mesenchymal transition-related proteins. Am J Dermatopathol. 2014;36(3):238–242. doi: 10.1097/DAD.0b013e3182987441.

[55] Terao M, Ishikawa A, Nakahara S, Kimura A, Kato A, Moriwaki K, Kamada Y, Murota H, Taniguchi N, Katayama I, Miyoshi E. Enhanced epithelial-mesenchymal transition-like phenotype in N-acetylglucosaminyltransferase V transgenic mouse skin promotes wound healing. J Biol Chem. 2011;286(32):28303–28311. doi: 10.1074/jbc.M111.220376.

[56] Sowalsky AG, Alt-Holland A, Shamis Y, Garlick JA, Feig LA. RalA function in dermal fibroblasts is required for the progression of squamous cell carcinoma of the skin. Cancer Res. 2011;71(3):758–767. doi: 10.1158/0008-5472.CAN-10-2756.

[57] Schlegel NC, von Planta A, Widmer DS, Dummer R, Christofori G. PI3K signalling is required for a TGFβ-induced epithelial-mesenchymal-like transition (EMT-like) in human melanoma cells. Exp Dermatol. 2015;24(1):22–28. doi: 10.1111/exd.12580.

[58] Lu X, Luo F, Liu Y, Zhang A, Li J, Wang B, Xu W, Shi L, Liu X, Lu L, Liu Q. The IL-6/STAT3 pathway via miR-21 is involved in the neoplastic and metastatic properties of arsenite-transformed human keratinocytes. Toxicol Lett. 2015;237(3):191–199. doi: 10.1016/j.toxlet.2015.06.011.

[59] Na YR, Lee JS, Lee SJ, Seok SH. Interleukin-6-induced Twist and N-cadherin enhance melanoma cell metastasis. Melanoma Res. 2013;23(6):434–443. doi: 10.1097/CMR.0000000000000021.

[60] Sou PW, Delic NC, Halliday GM, Lyons JG. Snail transcription factors in keratinocytes: enough to make your skin crawl. Int J Biochem Cell Biol. 2010;42(12):1940–1944. doi: 10.1016/j.biocel.2010.08.021.

[61] Byun JS, Gardner K. Wounds that will not heal: pervasive cellular reprogramming in cancer. Am J Pathol. 2013;182(4):1055–1064. doi: 10.1016/j.ajpath.2013.01.009.

[62] Li G, Satyamoorthy K, Herlyn M. Dynamics of cell interactions and communications during melanoma development. Crit Rev Oral Biol Med. 2002;13(1):62–70.

[63] Laidler P, Gil D, Pituch-Noworolska A, Ciołczyk D, Ksiazek D, Przybyło M, Lityńska A. Expression of beta1-integrins and N-cadherin in bladder cancer and melanoma cell lines. Acta Biochim Pol. 2000;47(4):1159–1170.

[64] Werling AM, Doerflinger Y, Brandner JM, Fuchs F, Becker JC, Schrama D, Kurzen H, Goerdt S, Peitsch WK. Homo- and heterotypic cell-cell contacts in Merkel cells and

Merkel cell carcinomas: heterogeneity and indications for cadherin switching. Histopathology. 2011;58(2):286–303. doi: 10.1111/j.1365-2559.2011.03748.x.

[65] Zhao P, Guo S, Tu Z, Di L, Zha X, Zhou H, Zhang X. Grhl3 induces human epithelial tumor cell migration and invasion via downregulation of E-cadherin. Acta Biochim Biophys Sin (Shanghai). 2016;48(3):266–274. doi: 10.1093/abbs/gmw001.

[66] Tang L, Yi XM, Chen J, Chen FJ, Lou W, Gao YL, Zhou J, Su LN, Xu X, Lu JQ, Ma J, Yu N, Ding YF. Ubiquitin ligase UBE3C promotes melanoma progression by increasing epithelial-mesenchymal transition in melanoma cells. Oncotarget. 2016;7(13):15738–15746. doi: 10.18632/oncotarget.7393.

[67] van Kempen LC, van den Hurk K, Lazar V, Michiels S, Winnepenninckx V, Stas M, Spatz A, van den Oord JJ. Loss of microRNA-200a and c, and microRNA-203 expression at the invasive front of primary cutaneous melanoma is associated with increased thickness and disease progression. Virchows Arch. 2012;461(4):441–448. doi: 10.1007/s00428-012-1309-9.

[68] Kreiseder B, Orel L, Bujnow C, Buschek S, Pflueger M, Schuett W, Hundsberger H, de Martin R, Wiesner C. α-Catulin downregulates E-cadherin and promotes melanoma progression and invasion. Int J Cancer. 2013;132(3):521–530. doi: 10.1002/ijc.27698.

[69] Knapp CF, Sayegh Z, Schell MJ, Rawal B, Ochoa T, Sondak VK, Messina JL. Expression of CXCR4, E-cadherin, Bcl-2, and survivin in Merkel cell carcinoma: an immunohistochemical study using a tissue microarray. Am J Dermatopathol. 2012;34(6):592–596. doi: 10.1097/DAD.0b013e31823e25d3.

[70] Shirley SH, Greene VR, Duncan LM, Torres Cabala CA, Grimm EA, Kusewitt DF. Slug expression during melanoma progression. Am J Pathol. 2012;180(6):2479–2489. doi: 10.1016/j.ajpath.2012.02.014.

[71] Wang Z, Liu L, Wang M, Shen M, Li J, Liu J, Li C, Xin C, Zhu S, Mei Q, Wang Y. NOTCH1 regulates migration and invasion of skin cancer cells by E-cadherin repression. Mol Cell Biochem. 2012;362(1–2):35–41. doi: 10.1007/s11010-011-1125-6.

[72] Alt-Holland A, Sowalsky AG, Szwec-Levin Y, Shamis Y, Hatch H, Feig LA, Garlick JA. Suppression of E-cadherin function drives the early stages of Ras-induced squamous cell carcinoma through upregulation of FAK and Src. J Invest Dermatol. 2011;131(11): 2306–2315. doi: 10.1038/jid.2011.188.

[73] Hao L, Ha JR, Kuzel P, Garcia E, Persad S. Cadherin switch from E- to N-cadherin in melanoma progression is regulated by the PI3K/PTEN pathway through Twist and Snail. Br J Dermatol. 2012;166(6):1184–1197. doi: 10.1111/j.1365-2133.2012.10824.x.

[74] Lade-Keller J, Riber-Hansen R, Guldberg P, Schmidt H, Hamilton-Dutoit SJ, Steiniche T. E- to N-cadherin switch in melanoma is associated with decreased expression of phosphatase and tensin homolog and cancer progression. Br J Dermatol. 2013;169(3): 618–628. doi: 10.1111/bjd.12426.

[75] Maretzky T, Reiss K, Ludwig A, Buchholz J, Scholz F, Proksch E, de Strooper B, Hartmann D, Saftig P. ADAM10 mediates E-cadherin shedding and regulates epithelial cell-cell adhesion, migration, and beta-catenin translocation. Proc Natl Acad Sci USA. 2005;102(26):9182–9187.

[76] Brouxhon SM, Kyrkanides S, Teng X, Athar M, Ghazizadeh S, Simon M, O'Banion MK, Ma L. Soluble E-cadherin: a critical oncogene modulating receptor tyrosine kinases, MAPK and PI3K/Akt/mTOR signaling. Oncogene. 2014;33(2):225–235. doi: 10.1038/onc.2012.563.

[77] Brouxhon SM, Kyrkanides S, Raja V, Silberfeld A, Teng X, Trochesset D, Cohen J, Ma L. Ectodomain-specific E-cadherin antibody suppresses skin SCC growth and reduces tumor grade: a multitargeted therapy modulating RTKs and the PTEN-p53-MDM2 axis. Mol Cancer Ther. 2014;13(7):1791–1802. doi: 10.1158/1535-7163.MCT-13-0971.

[78] George E, Polissar NL, Wick M. Immunohistochemical evaluation of p16INK4A, E-cadherin, and cyclin D1 expression in melanoma and Spitz tumors. Am J Clin Pathol. 2010;133(3):370–379. doi: 10.1309/AJCP52YVYCTLUOPI.

[79] Hsu M, Andl T, Li G, Meinkoth JL, Herlyn M. Cadherin repertoire determines partner-specific gap junctional communication during melanoma progression. J Cell Sci. 2000;113(9):1535–1542.

[80] Lin YS, Tsai PH, Kandaswami CC, Cheng CH, Ke FC, Lee PP, Hwang JJ, Lee MT. Effects of dietary flavonoids, luteolin, and quercetin on the reversal of epithelial-mesenchymal transition in A431 epidermal cancer cells. Cancer Sci. 2011;102(10):1829–1839. doi: 10.1111/j.1349-7006.2011.02035.x.

[81] Vieira AF, Paredes J. P-cadherin and the journey to cancer metastasis. Mol Cancer. 2015;14(1):178. doi: 10.1186/s12943-015-0448-4.

[82] Krengel S, Grotelüschen F, Bartsch S, Tronnier M. Cadherin expression pattern in melanocytic tumors more likely depends on the melanocyte environment than on tumor cell progression. J Cutan Pathol. 2004;31(1):1–7.

[83] Bauer R, Wild PJ, Meyer S, Bataille F, Pauer A, Klinkhammer-Schalke M, Hofstaedter F, Bosserhoff AK. Prognostic relevance of P-cadherin expression in melanocytic skin tumours analysed by high-throughput tissue microarrays. J Clin Pathol. 2006;59(7):699–705. doi: 10.1136/jcp.2005.034538.

[84] Bachmann IM, Straume O, Puntervoll HE, Kalvenes MB, Akslen LA. Importance of P-cadherin, beta-catenin, and Wnt5a/frizzled for progression of melanocytic tumors and prognosis in cutaneous melanoma. Clin Cancer Res. 2005;11(24 Pt 1):8606–8614. doi: 10.1158/1078-0432.CCR-05-0011

[85] Vlahova L, Doerflinger Y, Houben R, Becker JC, Schrama D, Weiss C, Goebeler M, Helmbold P, Goerdt S, Peitsch WK. P-cadherin expression in Merkel cell carcinomas is

associated with prolonged recurrence-free survival. Br J Dermatol. 2012;166(5):1043–1052. doi: 10.1111/j.1365-2133.2012.10853.x.

[86] DiVito KA, Trabosh VA, Chen YS, Chen Y, Albanese C, Javelaud D, Mauviel A, Simbulan-Rosenthal CM, Rosenthal DS. Smad7 restricts melanoma invasion by restoring N-cadherin expression and establishing heterotypic cell-cell interactions in vivo. Pigment Cell Melanoma Res. 2010;23(6):795–808. doi: 10.1111/j.1755-148X.2010.00758.x.

[87] Ciołczyk-Wierzbicka D, Gil D, Laidler P. The inhibition of cell proliferation using silencing of N-cadherin gene by siRNA process in human melanoma cell lines. Curr Med Chem. 2012;19(1):145–151.

[88] Zhou S, Matsuyoshi N, Liang SB, Takeuchi T, Ohtsuki Y, Miyachi Y. Expression of T-cadherin in basal keratinocytes of skin. J Invest Dermatol. 2002;118(6):1080–1084. doi: 10.1046/j.1523-1747.2002.01795.x.

[89] Kuphal S, Martyn AC, Pedley J, Crowther LM, Bonazzi VF, Parsons PG, Bosserhoff AK, Hayward NK, Boyle GM. H-cadherin expression reduces invasion of malignant melanoma. Pigment Cell Melanoma Res. 2009;22:296–306. doi: 10.1111/j.1755-148X.2009.00568.x.

[90] Bosserhoff AK, Ellmann L, Quast AS, Eberle J, Boyle GM, Kuphal S. Loss of T-cadherin (CDH-13) regulates AKT signaling and desensitizes cells to apoptosis in melanoma. Mol Carcinog. 2014;53:635–647. doi: 10.1002/mc.22018.

[91] Rubina KA, Yurlova EI, Sysoeva VY, Semina EV, Kalinina NI, Poliakov AA, Mikhaylova IN, Andronova NV, Treshalina HM. T-cadherin stimulates melanoma cell proliferation and mesenchymal stromal cell recruitment, but inhibits angiogenesis in a mouse melanoma model. In: Chai J, editor. Research Directions in Tumor Angiogenesis. Rijeka: InTechOpen; 2013, Chapter 6; p. 143–174. doi: 10.5772/53350

[92] Rubina KA, Surkova EI, Semina EV, Sysoeva VY, Kalinina NI, Poliakov AA, Treshalina HM, Tkachuk VA. T-cadherin expression in melanoma cells stimulates stromal cell recruitment and invasion by regulating the expression of chemokines, integrins and adhesion molecules. Cancers (Basels). 2015;7:1349–1370. doi: 10.3390/cancers7030840.

[93] Mukoyama Y, Zhou S, Miyachi Y, Matsuyoshi N. T-cadherin negatively regulates the proliferation of cutaneous squamous carcinoma cells. J Invest Dermatol. 2005;124:833–838. doi: 10.1111/j.0022-202X.2005.23660.x.

[94] Philippova M, Pfaff D, Kyriakakis E, Buechner SA, Iezzi G, Spagnoli GC,. Schoenenberger AW, Erne P, Resink TJ. T-cadherin loss promotes experimental metastasis of squamous cell carcinoma. Eur J Cancer. 2013;49:2048–2058. doi: 10.1016/j.ejca.2012.12.026.

[95] Zhou S, Matsuyoshi N, Takeuchi T, Ohtsuki Y, Miyachi Y. Reciprocal altered expression of T-cadherin and P-cadherin in psoriasis vulgaris. Br J Dermatol. 2003;149(2):268–273.

[96] Takeuchi T, Liang SB, Matsuyoshi N, Zhou S, Miyachi Y, Sonobe H, Ohtsuki Y. Loss of T-cadherin (CDH13, H-cadherin) expression in cutaneous squamous cell carcinoma. Lab Invest. 2002;82(8):1023–1029.

[97] Takeuchi T, Liang SB, Ohtsuki Y. Downregulation of expression of a novel cadherin molecule, T-cadherin, in basal cell carcinoma of the skin. Mol Carcinog. 2002A;35(4): 173–179. doi: 10.1002/mc.10088.

[98] Rubina K, Sysoeva V, Semina E, Kalinina N, Yurlova E, Khlebnikova A, Molochkov V. Malignant transformation in skin is associated with the loss of T-cadherin expression in human keratinocytes and heterogeneity in T-cadherin expression in tumor vasculature. In: Ran S, editor. Tumor Angiogenesis. Rijeka: InTechOpen; 2012, Chapter 6; p. 135–166. doi: 10.5772/26666

[99] Buechner SA, Philippova M, Erne P, Mathys T, Resink TJ. High T-cadherin expression is a feature of basal cell carcinoma. Br J Dermatol. 2009;161:199–201. doi: 10.1111/j. 1365-2133.2009.09195.x.

[100] Pfaff D, Philippova M, Buechner SA, Maslova K, Mathys T, Erne P, Resink TJ. T-cadherin loss induces an invasive phenotype in human keratinocytes and squamous cell carcinoma (SCC) cells in vitro and is associated with malignant transformation of cutaneous SCC in vivo. Br J Dermatol. 2010;163(2):353–363. doi: 10.1111/j. 1365-2133.2010.09801.x.

[101] Mukoyama Y, Utani A, Matsui S, Zhou S, Miyachi Y, Matsuyoshi N. T-cadherin enhances cell–matrix adhesiveness by regulating β1 integrin trafficking in cutaneous squamous carcinoma cells. Genes Cells. 2007;12:787–796. doi: 10.1111/j. 1365-2443.2007.01092.x.

[102] Kyriakakis E, Maslova K, Philippova M, Pfaff D, Joshi MB, Buechner SA, Erne P, Resink TJ. T-cadherin is an auxiliary negative regulator of EGFR pathway activity in cutaneous squamous cell carcinoma: Impact on cell motility. J Invest. Dermatol. 2012;132:2275–2285. doi: 10.1038/jid.2012.131.

[103] Neiva KG, Zhang Z, Miyazawa M, Warner KA, Karl E, Nör JE. Cross talk initiated by endothelial cells enhances migration and inhibits anoikis of squamous cell carcinoma cells through STAT3/Akt/ERK signaling. Neoplasia 2009;11(6):583–593.

[104] Kyriakakis E, Maslova K, Frachet A, Ferri N, Contini A, Pfaff D, Erne P, Resink TJ, Philippova M. Cross-talk between EGFR and T-cadherin: EGFR activation promotes T-cadherin localization to intercellular contacts. Cell Signall. 2013;25:1044–1053. doi: 10.1016/j.cellsig.2013.02.001.

[105] Siret C, Terciolo C, Dobric A, Habib MC, Germain S, Bonnier R, Lombardo D, Rigot V, André F. Interplay between cadherins and α2β1 integrin differentially regulates melanoma cell invasion. Br J Cancer. 2015;113(10):1445–1453. doi: 10.1038/bjc.2015.358.

[106] Perrais M, Chen X, Perez-Moreno M, Gumbiner BM. E-cadherin homophilic ligation inhibits cell growth and epidermal growth factor receptor signaling independently of

other cell interactions. Mol Biol Cell. 2007;18(6):2013–2025. doi: 10.1091/mbc.E06-04-0348.

[107] Lo HW, Hsu SC, Xia W, Cao X, Shih JY, Wei Y, Abbruzzese JL, Hortobagyi GN, Hung MC. Epidermal growth factor receptor cooperates with signal transducer and activator of transcription 3 to induce epithelial-mesenchymal transition in cancer cells via upregulation of TWIST gene expression. Cancer Res. 2007;67(19):9066–9076. doi: 10.1158/0008-5472.CAN-07-0575.

[108] Wang D, Su L, Huang D, Zhang H, Shin DM, Chen ZG. Downregulation of E-cadherin enhances proliferation of head and neck cancer through transcriptional regulation of EGFR. Mol Cancer. 2011;10:116. doi: 10.1186/1476-4598-10-116.

[109] Hazan RB, Norton L. The epidermal growth factor receptor modulates the interaction of E-cadherin with the actin cytoskeleton. J Biol Chem. 1998;273(15):9078–9084.

[110] Lobos-González L, Aguilar L, Diaz J, Diaz N, Urra H, Torres VA, Silva V, Fitzpatrick C, Lladser A, Hoek KS, Leyton L, Quest AF. E-cadherin determines Caveolin-1 tumor suppression or metastasis enhancing function in melanoma cells. Pigment Cell Melanoma Res. 2013;26(4):555–570. doi: 10.1111/pcmr.12085.

[111] Melo-Júnior MR, Araújo-Filho JLS, Ramos VJ, Patu M, de Paula Machado MCF, Beltrão EIC, Carvalho Jr LB. Digital image analysis of skin neoplasms evaluated by lectin histochemistry: potential marker to biochemical alterations and tumour differential diagnosis. Bras Patol Med Lab. 2006;42(6):455–460. doi: 10.1590/S1676-24442006000600009.

[112] Doré JF, Berthier-Vergnes O, Zebda N, Bailly M, Thomas L, Bailly C, Cochran AJ. Selective expression of PNA-binding glycoconjugates by invasive human melanomas: a new marker of metastatic potential. Pigment Cell Res. 1994;7(6):461–464.

[113] Lima LRA, Bezerra MF, Almeida SMV, Silva LPBG, Beltrão EIC, Carvalho Júnior LB. Glycophenotype evaluation in cutaneous tumors using lectins labeled with acridinium ester. Disease Markers. 2013;35(3):149–154. doi: 10.1155/2013/787130.

[114] Ferreira SA, Vasconcelos JLA, Cavalcanti LCB, Silva RCWC, Bezerra CL, Rêgo MJBM, Beltrão EIC. Expression patterns of α2,3-sialyltransferase I and α2,6-sialyltransferase I in human cutaneous epithelial lesions. Eur J Histochem. 2013;57:e7:41–45. doi: 10.4081/ejh.2013.e7.

[115] Sames K, Schumacher U, Halata Z, van Damme EJM, Peumans WJ, Asmus B, Moll R, Moll I. Lectin and proteoglycan histochemistry of Merkel cell carcinomas. Exp Dermatol. 2001;10:100–109.

[116] Varki A, Schauer R. Sialic acids. In: Varki A, Cummings RD, Esko JD, Freeze HH, Stanley P, Bertozzi CR, Hart GW, Etzler ME, editors. Essentials of Glycobiology. New York: Cold Spring Harbor Laboratory Press; 2009, Chapter 14.

[117] Nilsson LA, Gisslén H, Lindholm A, Lindholm L, Mobacken H. Identification of basal cell carcinomas by means of monoclonal antibodies C50 and C241. J Dermatol Surg Oncol. 1987;13(1):49–51.

[118] Thies A, Moll I, Berger J, Schumacher U. Lectin binding to cutaneous malignant melanoma: HPA is associated with metastasis formation. Br J Cancer. 2001;84(6):819–823. doi: 10.1054/bjoc.2000.1673.

[119] Thies A, Pfüller U, Schachner M, Horny HP, Molls I, Schumacher U. Binding of mistletoe lectins to cutaneous malignant melanoma: implications for prognosis and therapy. Anticancer Res. 2001;21(4B):2883–2887.

[120] Thies A, Berlin A, Brunner G, Schulze H-J, Moll I, Pfüller U, Wagener C, Schachner M, Altevogt P, Schumacher U. Glycoconjugate profiling of primary melanoma and its sentinel node and distant metastases: implications for diagnosis and pathophysiology of metastases. Can Lett. 2007;248:68–80. doi: 10.1016/j.canlet.2006.05.020.

[121] Carvalho S, Catarino TA, Dias AM, Kato M, Almeida A, Hessling B, Figueiredo J, Gärtner F, Sanches JM, Ruppert T, Miyoshi E, Pierce M, Carneiro F, Kolarich D, Seruca R, Yamaguchi Y, Taniguchi N, Reis CA, Pinho SS. Preventing E-cadherin aberrant N-glycosylation at Asn-554 improves its critical function in gastric cancer. Oncogene. 2016;35(13):1619–1631. doi: 10.1038/onc.2015.225.

[122] Guo HB, Johnson H, Randolph M, Pierce M. Regulation of homotypic cell-cell adhesion by branched N-glycosylation of N-cadherin extracellular EC2 and EC3 domains. J Biol Chem. 2009;284(50):34986–34997. doi: 10.1074/jbc.M109.060806.

[123] Adamczyk B, Tharmalingam T, Rudd PM. Glycans as cancer biomarkers. Biochim Biophys Acta. 2012;1820(9):1347–1353. doi: 10.1016/j.bbagen.2011.12.001.

[124] Janik ME, Lityńska A, Vereecken P. Cell migration—the role of integrin glycosylation. Biochim Biophys Acta. 2010;1800:545–555. doi: 10.1016/j.bbagen.2010.03.013.

[125] Yoshimura M, Ihara Y, Matsuzawa Y, Taniguchi N. Aberrant glycosylation of E-cadherin enhances cell-cell binding to suppress metastasis. J Biol Chem. 1996;271(23): 13811–13815.

[126] Lityńska A, Przybyło M, Pocheć E, Hoja-Łukowicz D, Ciołczyk D, Laidler P, Gil D. Comparison of the lectin-binding pattern in different human melanoma cell lines. Melanoma Res. 2001;11:1–8.

[127] Ciołczyk-Wierzbicka D, Gil D, Hoja-Łukowicz D, Lityńska A, Laidler P. Carbohydrate moieties of N-cadherin from human melanoma cell lines. Acta Biochim Pol. 2002;49(4): 991–998. doi: 024904991.

[128] Przybyło M, Martuszewska D, Pocheć E, Hoja-Łukowicz D, Lityńska A. Identification of proteins bearing beta1-6 branched N-glycans in human melanoma cell lines from different progression stages by tandem mass spectrometry analysis. Biochim Biophys Acta. 2007;1770(9):1427–1435. doi: 10.1016/j.bbagen.2007.05.006.

[129] Zhu W, Leber B, Andrews DW. Cytoplasmic O-glycosylation prevents cell surface transport of E-cadherin during apoptosis. EMBO J. 2001;20:5999–6007. doi: 10.1093/emboj/20.21.5999.

[130] Ciołczyk-Wierzbicka D, Amoresano A, Casbarra A, Hoja-Łukowicz D, Lityńska A, Laidler P. The structure of the oligosaccharides of N-cadherin from human melanoma cell lines. Glycoconj J. 2004;20(7–8):483–492. doi: 10.1023/B:GLYC.0000038294.72088.b0.

Section 4

Metabolism

Chapter 6

Inhibiting Lactate Dehydrogenase A Enhances the Cytotoxicity of the Mitochondria Accumulating Antioxidant, Mitoquinone, in Melanoma Cells

Ali A. Alshamrani, James L. Franklin,
Aaron M. Beedle and Mandi M. Murph

Additional information is available at the end of the chapter

http://dx.doi.org/10.5772/64231

Abstract

Limited options exist for inhibitors targeted against melanoma tumors with mutation subtypes other than BRAF. We investigated the cytotoxic activity of mitoquinone (MitoQ), an antioxidant and ubiquinone derivative, on various human melanoma cell lines, alone or in combination with other agents to perturb cellular bioenergetics. This lipophilic cation crosses the cell membrane, enters and accumulates in the mitochondria where it can disrupt mitochondrial function at micromolar concentrations or act as an antioxidant to preserve membrane integrity at nanomolar concentrations. Consistent with previous studies, cells treated with 12.5 μM MitoQ show significantly reduced viability versus control treatments. Although all melanoma cells were susceptible to cytotoxicity induced by MitoQ, cells with wild-type BRAF were responsive to lower doses, compared to cells with activating mutations in BRAF. Mechanistically, the positively charged lipophilic moiety of the MitoQ induced a dose-dependent collapse of the mitochondrial membrane potential ($\Delta\psi m$) and significantly reduced the mitochondrial ATP production and reduced oxygen consumption rate, suggesting mitochondrial dysfunction. We also combined MitoQ with a glycolytic lactate dehydrogenase A inhibitor (FX-11) and observed an enhanced reduction in viability, but not other therapies examined. To summarize, the data suggest that FX-11 enhances the cytotoxic effects of MitoQ in cells with wild-type BRAF.

Keywords: MitoQ, BRAF, dTPP, melanoma, cytotoxicity

1. Introduction

Mitoquinone (MitoQ) is a synthetic compound and functional antioxidant that enters the mitochondria and accumulates there. Low doses thwart lipid peroxidation, whereas doses above 1 μM can disrupt mitochondria membrane integrity [1, 2]. MitoQ has a ubiquinone moiety covalently connected through a 10-carbon alkyl chain to a lipophilic cation triphenylphosphonium (TPP+) moiety [3, 4]. Recently, this TPP+ moiety has also been shown to inhibit the mitochondrial electron transport chain and induce mitochondrial proton leak [5].

However, additional molecular mechanisms by which these lipophilic cations induce antitumorigenic effects likely exist. Previously, such mitochondria-targeted lipophilic cations displayed cytotoxic activity against hepatocellular carcinoma and breast cancer using cell culture and/or animal models of malignancy [6–8]. Unfortunately, controversy surrounds whether MitoQ can be utilized to prevent age-associated diseases, since some clinical trials showed a lack of efficacy in models outside of cancer [9, 10].

The mitochondria are the cell's powerhouse, responsible for the production of adenosine triphosphate (ATP), the energy required by the cell, utilizing a process called oxidative phosphorylation. Although mechanisms of aerobic cellular respiration are far more efficient in the production of ATP, many tumorigenic cells curiously switch to anaerobic metabolism (glycolysis) during malignant transformation, despite the presence of oxygen, which can be referred to as the "Warburg effect" [11]. This abnormal reprogramming of energy metabolism is therefore a hallmark of cancer [12]. However, not all cancer cells utilize glycolysis, which provides far less ATP, but at a much faster rate. At least prostate and breast cancers, as well as leukemias, likely require oxidative phosphorylation [13].

Intriguingly, studies also suggest that melanoma cells are dependent upon oxidative phosphorylation and show significantly more oxygen consumption than their normal counterparts, the melanocytes [13]. Alternatively, other studies suggest that melanoma cells may vacillate between utilizing either oxidative phosphorylation or glycolysis, depending on the environmental conditions [14]. Since cells found within tumors are highly heterogenic, it is likely that both conditions could be found at different locations when sampling the same tumor specimen.

Malignant cells reprogram or vacillate their cellular metabolism to meet the anabolic requirements for growth and proliferation while also sustaining their survival and viability amid harsh microenvironments with limited nutrients [15]. Among melanoma cells, this bioenergetic switch has been suggested to be a direct consequence of an oncogenic activating mutation in BRAF [13]. This further insinuates that melanomas expressing wild-type BRAF versus mutant BRAF proteins would respond differently to compounds that target the mitochondria. Since 2011, the armamentarium has grown tremendously for small molecule inhibitors targeting BRAF melanomas, including vemurafenib, cobimetinib, dabrafenib, and trametinib, but there is a lack of targeted therapeutics for those cancer subtypes without the BRAF mutation.

In this study, we sought to investigate whether MitoQ has cytotoxic activity against human melanoma cell lines, both wild-type and BRAF mutant melanomas, alone or in combination with other agents to perturb cellular bioenergetics. We observed that cells treated with MitoQ have significantly less viability than controls and display enhanced mitochondrial dysfunction due to a decrease in mitochondrial metabolism. Our results also demonstrate that the cytotoxic effect was mediated by the positively charged lipophilic moiety of the MitoQ, since (1-Decyl)triphenylphosphonium bromide (dTPP) recapitulated the reduction in cell viability. Furthermore, we found that MitoQ displayed lower IC_{50} when combined with the FX-11, a small molecule that inhibits lactate dehydrogenase A, compared to single agent treatment.

2. Materials and methods

2.1. Cell culture

BRAF wild-type (MeWo) and *BRAF* mutant (A375) human melanoma cell lines were originally purchased from the American Type Culture Collection (ATCC®, Manassas, VA). *BRAF* wild-type (SB-2) and *BRAF* mutant (SK-MEL-5) human melanoma cell lines were obtained from The University of Texas MD Anderson Cancer Center (Houston, TX) and the National Cancer Institute NCI/NIH (Frederick, MD), respectively. All cell culture materials were purchased from Life Technologies®, Thermo Fisher Scientific Inc. (Waltham, MA). SB-2 and SK-MEL-5 cells were grown in DMEM while MeWo and A375 cells were grown in Roswell Park Memorial Institute (RPMI 1640) medium supplemented with 5% fetal bovine serum, or without for serum-free medium, and 1% penicillin/streptomycin was used to culture and maintain cell lines (Gibco® and Thermo Fisher Scientific Inc.). Cells were cultured at 37°C in an atmosphere of 95% humidity and 5% CO_2. The medium was changed every 48 h. Cells were maintained for at least three subsequent passages after thawing prior to conducting the experiments to ensure the stability of their physiochemical properties. For the no-glucose media, we used RPMI 1640 deprived of glucose and HEPES buffer (Invitrogen®, Carlsbad, CA) that contained 2 mM L-glutamine and was supplemented with 5% FBS and 1% penicillin/streptomycin. For the high-glucose media, we used no-glucose media (above) supplemented with 25 mM glucose. For the galactose media, we used no-glucose media (above) supplemented with 10 mM galactose. The 100 mM glucose and galactose stock solutions were prepared by dissolving 1.8016 g of glucose or galactose powders into a 50 mL deionized water, volume to 100 mL, and then either sterilized by autoclaving (glucose solution) or filtration (galactose solution) to make it suitable for cell culturing purposes.

2.2. Chemicals

The mitochondrial antioxidant MitoQ was kindly provided by Dr. Michael P. Murphy, Medical Research Council Mitochondrial Biology Unit, Cambridge, United Kingdom, to J.L.F. Chemotherapeutic agents cis-Diamineplatinum(II) dichloride and dacarbazine were purchased from Sigma-Aldrich® (St Louis, MO). The lipophilic cation (1-Decyl)triphenylphosphonium bromide (dTPP) was purchased from Santa Cruz Biotechnology® (Dallas, TX). The LPA1/3 receptor antagonist, Ki16425 was purchased from Selleck® Chemicals (Houston, TX). The autotaxin inhibitors HA-130 and PF-8380, along with the lactate dehydrogenase A inhibitor

FX-11 were purchased from Calbiochem®/EMD Millipore (Billerica, MA). The oxidative stress and apoptosis inducer elesclomol was purchased from ApexBio® Technology LLC (Houston, TX).

2.3. Cell viability assay

MeWo, SB-2, SK-MEL-5, and A375 cells were seeded into standard, flat-bottom, clear 96-well plates at 5000–10,000 cells per well. Twenty-four hours after seeding, cells were maintained in either high glucose or galactose media for 48 h as previously described [16]. For drug treatments, compound stock solutions were prepared in distilled water (MitoQ, dTPP, Ki16425) or dimethyl sulfoxide (DMSO – cisplatin, DTIC, Elesclomol, FX-11, HA-130, and PF-8380), and then added to the wells to give the final drug concentrations (ranging from 0.1 to 200 μM) using different conditioned media where indicated. Cells were then incubated for 24 h and cell viability was measured using the CellTiter-Blue® viability assay Promega (Madison, WI) as previously described [17–20]. For combination experiments, MeWo cells were treated with the IC_{50} of FX-11, HA-130 or PF-8380 in combination with increasing concentrations of the MitoQ (0.8–50 μM) and incubated for 24 h in serum-free medium.

2.4. Mitochondrial toxicity assay

MeWo cells were plated at 5000 cells/well on standard, flat-bottom, clear 96-well plates with a final media volume of 100 μL/well. After 24 h, cells were then maintained in either high glucose or galactose media for 48 h as previously described prior to treatment with different compounds. Cells were then treated with MitoQ at different concentrations ranging from 1 to 200 μM in different conditioned media as specified above. In addition, cells were treated with a positive control toxic compound, digitonin (200 μM) and then both groups were incubated for 3 h at 37°C in an atmosphere of 95% humidity and 5% CO_2. Cellular toxicity profiles were generated using the Mitochondrial ToxGlo™ Assay Promega (Madison, WI) following the manufacturer's protocol. Next, an ATP detection reagent that consists of luciferin, ATPase inhibitors, and thermostable Ultra-Glo™ luciferase was utilized to lyse viable cells and assess their ATP levels. This combination of reagents generates a luminescent signal proportional to the amount of ATP present.

2.5. Oxygen consumption rate assay

MeWo cells were seeded at 15,000 cells/well on standard, flat-bottom, clear 96-well plates, and incubated for 24 h. Cells were treated with increasing concentrations of MitoQ (6.25–100 μM) for 20 min prior to the assessment of cellular respiration using Oxygen Consumption Rate Assay Kit MitoXpress®-Xtra HS Method, Cayman Chemicals (Ann Arbor, MI) following the manufacturer's protocol. The phosphorescent oxygen probe provided by the kit is quenched by oxygen in the extracellular medium. Therefore, the signal intensity obtained using this kit is proportional to the increase in the oxygen consumption rate by cells.

2.6. Assessment of the mitochondrial membrane potential (Δψm)

MeWo cells were plated at 3000 cells/well in standard, flat-bottom, clear 96-well plates, and incubated for 24 h. Cells were washed twice with warm phosphate buffered saline and the nuclei were stained using NucBlue® live cell Hoechst 33342 stain following the manufacturer's protocol. Cells were then washed one time with warm PBS and then incubated in warm live cell imaging solution containing 20 nM tetramethylrhodamine methyl ester (TMRM) dye (Molecular Probes™, Thermo Fisher Scientific) for 30 min in the dark at room temperature prior to the treatment with MitoQ (12.5–100 μM) or left untreated. Fluorescent imaging was performed to visualize nuclear (Hoechst) and mitochondrial (TMRM) staining with DAPI and TRITC filters, respectively, using an X71 inverted fluorescent microscope (Olympus, Center Valley, PA).

2.7. Fluorescence images analysis

MeWo cells were viewed using an Olympus X71 inverted epifluorescent microscope (40× objective) with an ND25 neutral density filter and images were captured using a DP-72 camera with identical black balance correction and exposure time in the CellSens Software (Olympus). Fluorescence microscopy experiments were repeated three times and three random pictures per condition per experiment were used to quantify the TMRM dye fluorescence intensity ($n = 3$) using Image-Pro® Insight 8.0 (MediaCybernetics®, Rockville, MD). The TMRM corrected fluorescence intensity was calculated for each image by normalizing the total red fluorescence of each entire 40× image (total TMRM intensity) by the number of cells in the same image (determined by the number of DAPI nuclei counted by manual tag in Image-Pro® Insight) to eliminate the impact of the differences in cell numbers between wells on our interpretation of data. Cells per image ranged from 135 to 270. Average TMRM corrected intensities for each dosing condition were expressed as relative percentage of the fluorescence intensities of untreated cells.

2.8. Statistical analysis

The statistical differences in experimental data were analyzed using analysis of variance (ANOVA) test, followed by either Tukey's or Bonferroni's multiple comparisons tests between groups using GraphPad Prism (La Jolla, CA). Student's *t*-test was used when only two groups are compared. $^{*}p < 0.05$, $^{**}p < 0.01$, and $^{***}p < 0.001$ indicate the levels of significance.

3. Results

To study the cytotoxic effects of the mitochondria-targeted lipophilic cation MitoQ in melanoma cells, we treated BRAF wild-type melanoma cells, MeWo and SB-2, or melanoma cells with *BRAF* activating mutations, A375 or SK-MEL-5, with increasing concentrations of MitoQ (0.8–50 μM) for 24 h (white bars) or 48 h (red bars). The data suggest that incubation with MitoQ during this period significantly suppresses the viability all cell lines in a dose-dependent manner (**Figure 1A**). Notably, MeWo and SB-2 cells are more sensitive to lower concentrations of MitoQ (0.8–12.5 μM at 24 h; $p < 0.001$), when compared to A375 or SK-MEL-5 cells (**Figure 1B**). We assessed cell viability 24 h posttreatment in MeWo cells with increasing concentrations (0.8–200 μM) of cisplatin, dacarbazine, Ki16425, PF-8380, and HA-130 and elesclomol to evaluate the cytotoxic potency of MitoQ in comparison with other chemotherapeutics (as negative controls) or investigational compounds (**Figure 1C**). MitoQ significantly affected cell viability at lower concentrations (3.1–50 μM) in MeWo cells when compared with other agents ($^{*}p < 0.05$).

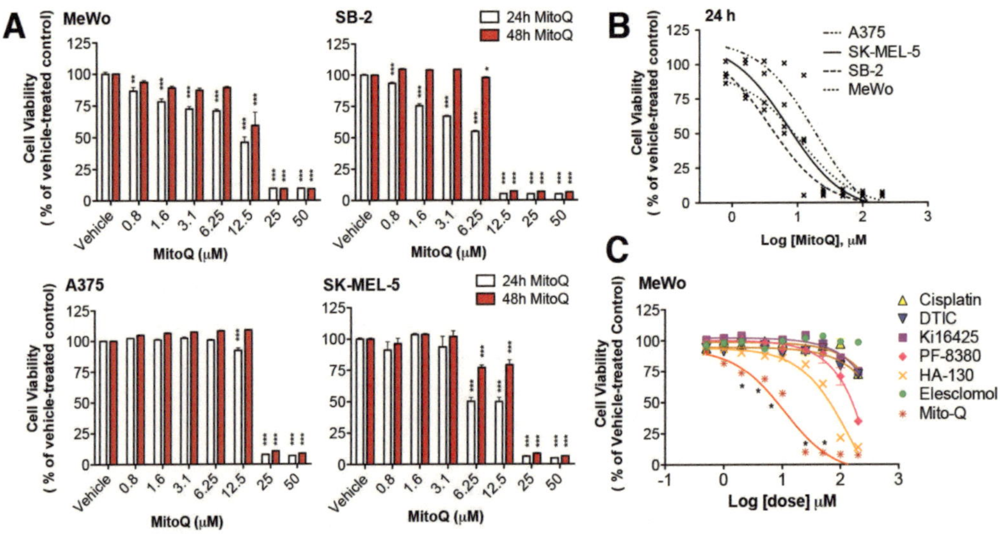

Figure 1. The viability of melanoma cells is significantly impacted after MitoQ treatment. To evaluate the potential cytotoxic effects of MitoQ in melanoma cells, (A) *BRAF* wild-type cells, MeWo and SB-2, or *BRAF* mutant cells, A375 and SK-MEL-5, were treated with increasing concentrations for 24 h (white bars) or 48 h (red bars) prior to determining cell viability. The data are expressed as the percentage of vehicle-treated controls (set at 100%) within each experiment and the mean ± SEM, $n = 3$ per treatment group ($^{**}p < 0.01$; $^{***}p < 0.001$) indicate significant differences between vehicle versus treatment conditions. (B) The 24 h treatment data are also presented in logarithmic scale as a comparison between cell lines. (C) To assess the cytotoxicity of MitoQ in comparison with other approved drugs or investigational compounds, MeWo cells were treated with increasing concentrations (0.8–50 μM) for 24 h prior to the assessment of viability.

Since MeWo cells are more sensitive to MitoQ treatment than A375 or SK-MEL-5 cells, we used MeWo cells to examine whether the MitoQ-induced cytotoxicity of melanoma cells is resultant from dysfunctional mitochondria. For this assay, cells were treated with increasing concentrations (0.8–200 μM) of MitoQ in the presence of high glucose or glucose-deprived/galactose-supplemented medium. Replacing glucose with galactose in the medium is a well-established approach to study the effect of mitochondrial toxins in cancer cells [16, 21–23]. The purpose of this switch is to augment the susceptibility of cells to the MitoQ-mediated mitochondrial toxicity. Indeed, replacing glucose with galactose significantly exacerbates the cytotoxic effects of MitoQ after 24 or 48 h of treatment (**Figure 2A**). As a correlative, we measured the intracellular ATP levels after a 3 h treatment with increasing concentrations of MitoQ. MeWo cells cultured in galactose-supplemented medium exhibited significant reduction (***$p < 0.001$) among intracellular ATP levels with MitoQ treatment (**Figure 2B**).

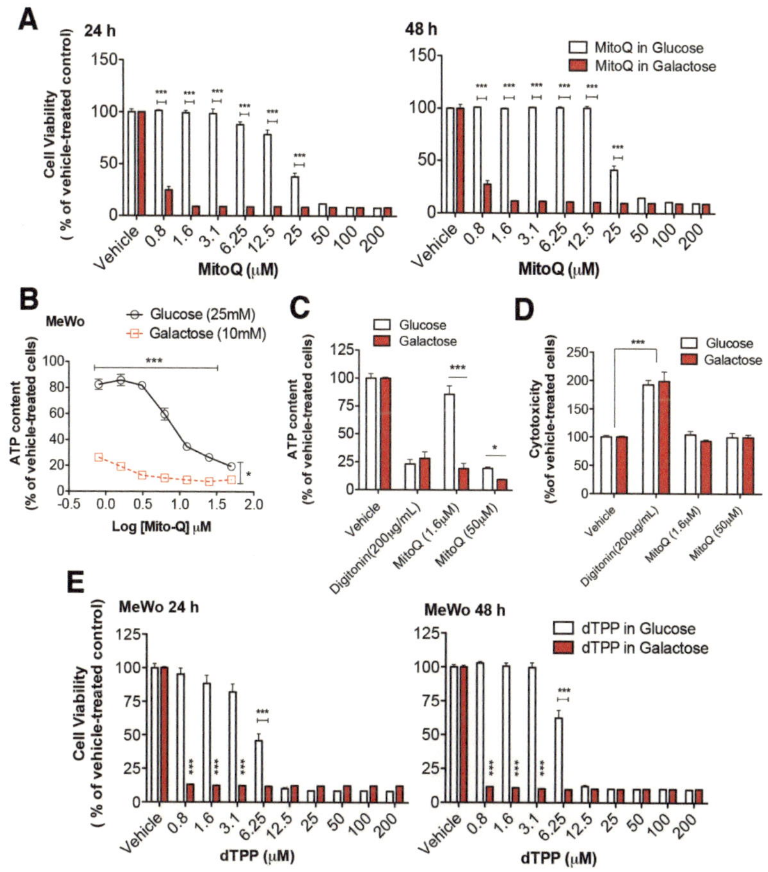

Figure 2. Replacing cell culture medium containing glucose with galactose increases susceptibility to MitoQ-mediated cytotoxicity. To determine whether the MitoQ-induced cytotoxicity is the result of dysfunctional mitochondria, we maintained MeWo cells in high glucose (25 mM) or galactose (10 mM)-supplemented medium for (A) 24 or 48 h prior to MitoQ treatment. Cells cultured in galactose-supplemented media rely on the mitochondria to generate ATP and sustain viability, which make them more suitable to mitochondrial toxicants. (B) ATP levels of MeWo cells were measured using ToxGlo™ Assay after 3 h exposure to increasing concentrations of MitoQ with cells cultured in different medium. (C) Results are also shown as the percentage of vehicle-treated controls (set at 100%) within experiments using the indicated concentrations of MitoQ or digitonin. (D) Plasma membrane cytotoxicity was assessed using the indicated concentrations of MitoQ or digitonin. (E) The viability of MeWo cells was measured in the presence of dTPP with cells cultured in either glucose (black bars) or galactose (red bars) for 24 or 48 h as indicated. Data are expressed as means ± SEM, $n = 3$ per treatment group. *$p < 0.05$ and ***$p < 0.001$ indicate significant differences between groups.

We then assessed the cell membrane integrity using a fluorogenic peptide substrate (bis-AAF-R110) that measures dead-cell protease activity. This peptide cannot cross the intact cell membranes of live cells and, therefore, the fluorescence signal is proportional to the non-live cells with compromised cell membranes. MitoQ treatment did not change cell membrane integrity in conditioned medium, unlike the cytotoxic compound digitonin, which is a detergent that can dissolve cell membranes, block ATP production, and subsequently cause cell death. Here, the positive control digitonin caused a significant reduction in ATP (**Figure 2C**) and a twofold change in the cell membrane integrity (**Figure 2D**). Taken together, these data suggest that the cytotoxicity mediated via MitoQ potently affects mitochondria; however, it does not indicate the moiety responsible. Thus, we treated cells with dTPP, the positively charged lipophilic cation contained within the structure of MitoQ. Indeed, cells in galactose-containing medium were not viable in the presence of 0.8 μM dTPP at 24 or 48 h (**Figure 2E**), suggesting this component is responsible for the MitoQ-induced cytotoxicity.

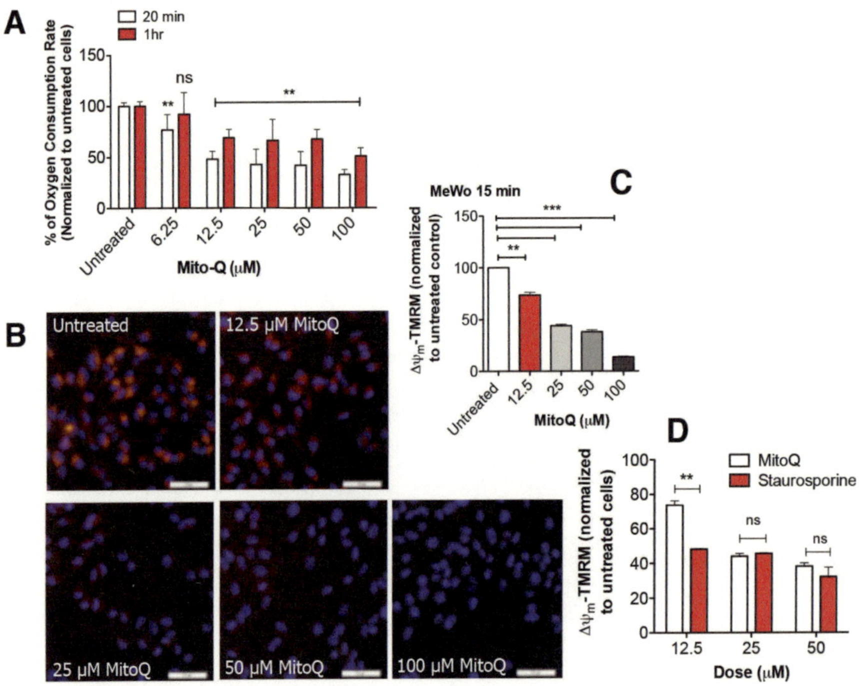

Figure 3. MitoQ induces a dose-dependent reduction in the mitochondrial transmembrane potential in melanoma cells. (A) The oxygen consumption rate was measured in untreated or MeWo cells treated with increasing concentrations of MitoQ for 20 min (white bars) or 1 h (red bars). (B) Representative fluorescence microscopic images of MeWo cells are shown after staining with TMRM (20 nM) and nuclear DAPI stain in the absence or presence of MitoQ (12.5, 25, 50, and 100 μM). (C) The bar graph shows quantification of TMRM signals after incubation for 30 min followed by 15 min treatment with MitoQ. The intensity of TMRM reflects the level of mitochondrial transmembrane potential, which indicate functional respiratory chain complexes. Treating MeWo cells with MitoQ resulted in a significant, dose-dependent reduction in the mitochondrial transmembrane potential, further suggesting mitochondrial dysfunction. (D) The bar graph shows TMRM intensity of MitoQ-treated cells is compared to staurosporine treatments. All data are expressed as mean ± SEM. Scale bar: 50 μm. $^{**}p < 0.01$, $^{***}p < 0.001$ indicate a significant difference between MitoQ treated and untreated cells.

To further confirm this mechanism, we measured the oxygen consumption rate of MeWo cells in response to acute exposure. The data show that MitoQ (20 min to 1 h) causes a significant reduction in the respiratory capacity of the mitochondria (**Figure 3A**). In addition, we assessed the impact of MitoQ on the mitochondrial membrane potential (Δψm) using fluorescent

TMRM dye, which reflects the level of mitochondrial transmembrane potential—an indication of functional respiratory chain complexes. Data show the dose-dependent (**Figure 3B**) and rapid (15 min) collapse (**Figure 3C**) of the mitochondrial membrane potential (Δψm) in treated MeWo cells. Unlike staurosporine, the potent protein kinase inhibitor that is cytotoxic to mammalian tumor cell lines, which induced an apparent maximal reduction in the Δψm at different concentrations (12.5–50 μM), MitoQ caused a dose-dependent collapse of the Δψm (**Figure 3D**). These data show that MitoQ disrupted the mitochondrial respiratory chain and oxidative phosphorylation prior to decreases in cell viability, suggesting that these events lead to the subsequent melanoma cell cytotoxicity.

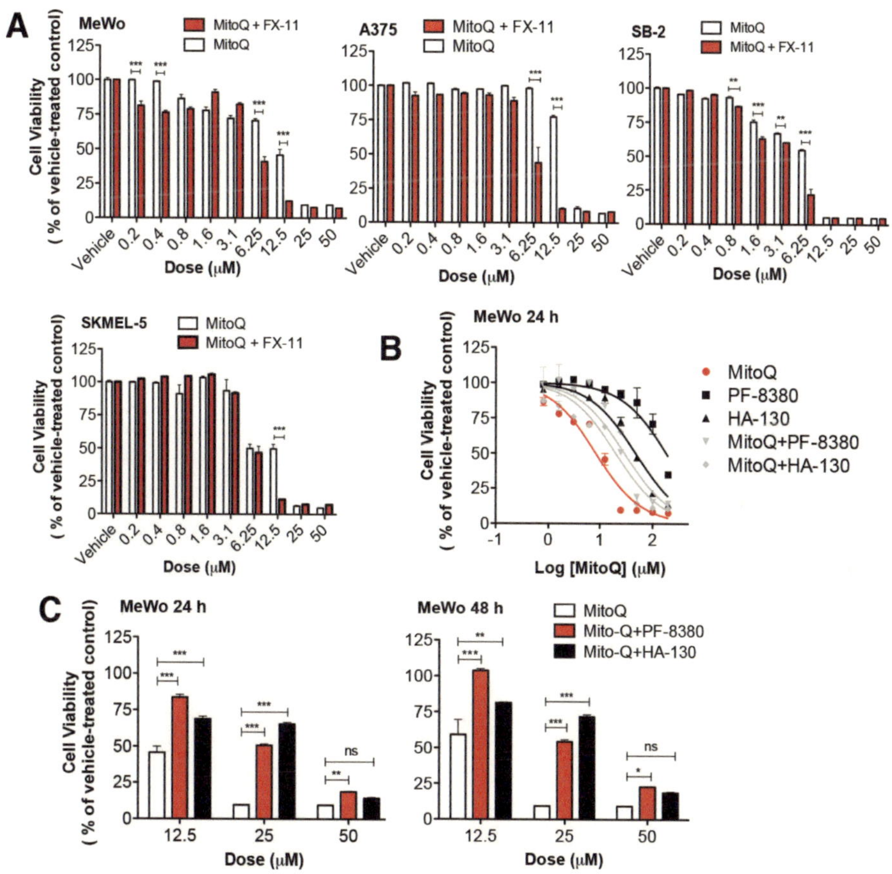

Figure 4. Inhibiting lactate dehydrogenase A enhances the cytotoxicity induced by MitoQ in melanoma cells. (A) MeWo, A375, SB-2, and SK-MEL-5 cells were treated with increasing concentrations of MitoQ for 24 h in the absence (white bars) and presence (red bars) of the lactate dehydrogenase inhibitor (FX-11, 5 μM). (B) Treatment of MeWo cells with 24 h MitoQ in combination with the autotaxin inhibitors, PF-8380 and HA-130 reduces, rather than enhances, the cytotoxic effects of MitoQ. (C) The viability of MeWo cells treated with the highest concentrations (12.5, 25, and 50 μM) of MitoQ alone or in combination with different autotaxin inhibitors for 24 and 48 h are shown. Cell viability is shown as percentage of vehicle-treated controls (set at 100%) within all experiments. Data shown represent the mean ± SEM, $n = 3$ per treatment group. $^{*}p < 0.05$, $^{**}p < 0.01$, and $^{***}p < 0.001$ indicate significant differences between single and combination therapies.

Since melanoma cells can reprogram their metabolism toward aerobic glycolysis to survive in case of mitochondrial dysfunction, we hypothesized that inhibition of the lactate dehydrogenase A (LDHA) enzyme would force the cells to rely on the mitochondria. Thus, this would increase vulnerability to MitoQ-induced cytotoxicity. Indeed, inhibition of LDHA using FX-11 enhanced the cytotoxic effects of MitoQ among MeWo, A375, SB-2, and SK-MEL-5 cells after 24 h of incubation (**Figure 4A**). Interestingly, the combination of MitoQ with investigational autotaxin inhibitors PF-8380 and HA-130 for 24 h reduced, rather than enhanced, the cytotoxic capabilities of MitoQ (**Figure 4B**). The significant difference among treated groups is clearly demonstrated at 12.5 and 25 μM (**Figure 4C**). The IC_{50} values further reflect the increase in cytotoxicity with combinations between MitoQ and FX-11 against other comparisons (**Table 1**). These data suggest that disruption of the cellular metabolic machinery serves as a potential cytotoxic strategy against melanoma *in vitro* and warrants further investigation *in vivo*.

Cell line	MitoQ Ave IC_{50} (μM) 24 h	MitoQ 95% CI	MitoQ + FX-11 Ave IC_{50} (μM) 24 h	MitoQ + FX-11 95% CI
MeWo	8.415	6.826–10.37	4.957	3.559–6.905
SB-2	5.152	2.694–9.856	2.876	2.041–4.052
A375	18.44	8.302–40.96	4.594	2.196–9.615
SK-MEL-5	10.67	4.666–24.39	1.344	0.6846–2.638
Cell line	**MitoQ Ave IC_{50} (μM) 48 h**	**MitoQ 95% CI**	**MitoQ + FX-11 Ave IC_{50} (μM) 48 h**	**MitoQ + FX-11 95% CI**
MeWo	13.08	9.371–18.02	8.009	5.252–12.21
SB-2	11.01	3.683–32.88	6.505	3.194–13.25
A375	21.41	8.534–53.70	5.284	2.359–11.83
SK-MEL-5	26.04	9.498–71.40	7.327	4.251–12.63

Table 1. Cell viability IC_{50} values after 24 or 48 h of treatment with MitoQ and FX-11.

4. Discussion

The data suggest that melanoma cells are susceptible to cytotoxicity mediated by the functional antioxidant, MitoQ, by inducing a dose-dependent reduction in the basal oxygen consumption rate and a rapid depolarization of the mitochondrial membrane potential. Culturing MeWo cells in galactose-supplemented medium significantly reduces intracellular ATP levels in response to MitoQ treatment, compared with culturing in glucose-containing medium. The data show that MitoQ did not affect the plasma membrane integrity, unlike the cell membrane permeabilizing compound, digitonin. Importantly, our study demonstrates that dual disruption of the metabolic machinery enhances the cytotoxicity of MitoQ using FX-11 (**Figure 5**).

The ability of cancer cells, melanoma cells in particular, to reprogram their metabolism has emerged as a major factor that leads to the development of resistance to many existing therapeutics [15, 24]. Recent studies have demonstrated that high levels of lactate dehydrogenase (LDH), an enzyme that converts the cytosolic pyruvate into lactate, could be utilized as a predictor of disease progression and chemotherapy response in addition to its involvement in the resistance of different types of cancer cells, including melanoma cells to chemotherapeutic drugs [25, 26]. Results from a recent Phase III clinical trial revealed that metastatic melanoma patients with high serum levels of LDH have shown less favorable responses to elesclomol, a promising first-in-class mitochondria-targeted compound that exerts anticancer activity by inducing oxidative stress and subsequent apoptotic cell death [27].

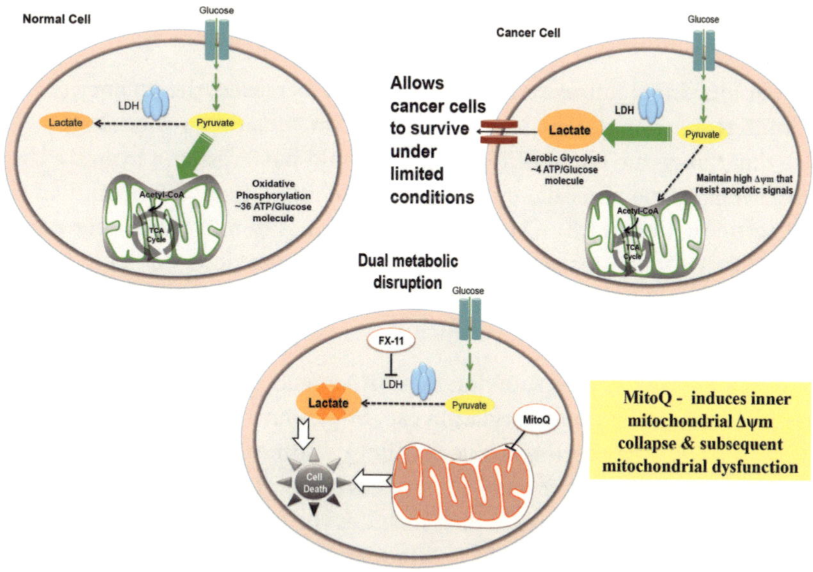

Figure 5. Working model of the observed treatment effects. This schematic illustration represents how targeting lactate metabolism enhances the cytotoxic effects of the mitochondria-targeted lipophilic cation MitoQ in melanoma cells. The normal cell depicted here is generating ATP through mitochondrial oxidative phosphorylation. During malignant transformation, cancer cells tend to strategically reprogram their metabolism toward aerobic glycolysis to produce lactate in order to acidify the surrounding tumor microenvironment and to survive in the harsh and metabolically limiting conditions, which is illustrated here by the cancer cell. In addition, the cancer cell is also maintaining functional mitochondria to resist apoptotic signals. The bottom cell shows our working model with dual disruption of metabolic machinery using a combination of MitoQ and FX-11 to counteract the melanoma cell's viability.

Therefore, we hypothesized that inhibiting cellular aerobic glycolysis would create a synergistic response to the cytotoxic effects of MitoQ, an approach conducted by several studies whereby mitochondria-targeted compounds were used in combination with glycolysis inhibitor, 2-deoxyglucose (2-DG). However, due to the high concentration of 2-DG needed to achieve the desirable synergistic cancer cell growth arrest [7, 8, 28], we were eager to find a more potent and irreversible glycolysis inhibitor that could augment MitoQ's cytotoxicity. Thus, in this study we found that the cytotoxic effects of MitoQ were synergistically enhanced when combined with a subtoxic (5 μM) concentration of FX-11, a selective suppressor of lactate dehydrogenase A. These data suggest that FX-11-treated cells were forced to rely more on mitochondrial oxidative phosphorylation to survive, which made them more vulnerable to the effects of the lipophilic cation MitoQ.

Recently, Trnka et al. have shown that longer aliphatic chains that link the positively charged triphenylphosphonium with any biologically active compound to target mitochondria inhibited the mitochondrial electron transport chain and induced mitochondrial proton leak [5]. Herein we observed that the MitoQ-induced cytotoxicity was mediated by the lipophilic cation dTPP moiety of MitoQ, rather than the redox cycling of the antioxidant moiety (ubiquinone). If dTPP is more potent than MitoQ, this is suggestive that the ubiquinone moiety may be protecting against the toxic effect of dTPP. Lastly, our results are in agreement with other publications [3, 5] showing the massive mitochondrial accumulation of the lipophilic cation moiety disrupts cellular respiratory capacities and induces cytotoxicity.

Surprisingly, autotaxin inhibitors reduced, rather than increased, the potency of MitoQ. Since autotaxin inhibitors have shown superior activity in melanoma models [18, 20, 29], we hypothesize that this reduction in MitoQ potency could have resulted from the disruption of mitochondrial membrane potential by autotaxin inhibitors. If so, this would affect the integration and accumulation of MitoQ into the mitochondria of melanoma cells and reduce the compound's efficacy. Our observation is in agreement with previous studies in which autotaxin has been reported to protect breast cancer and melanoma cells against Taxol-induced cell death through maintaining their mitochondrial membrane potential [30].

Consistent with previous studies showing that BRAF wild-type cells, including MeWo cells, display enhanced oxidative phosphorylation capabilities and mitochondrial capacity [31], we observed that these cells are more sensitive to MitoQ treatment than A375 cells, which possess an activating BRAF mutation. Therefore, our study is relevant to developing targeted strategies against wild-type BRAF melanomas, which includes the subtypes RAS, NF1, and Triple-WT [32], with the most relevance to Triple-WT. Although the majority of melanoma patients have tumors with activating mutations in BRAF, and thus are candidates for BRAF inhibitors like vemurafenib, trametinib, dabrafenib, and cobimetinib, those patients that have tumors with wild-type BRAF lack a clear strategy for targeted therapy. BRAF status of melanoma cells has been directly linked to cellular metabolism and the bioenergetic switch between mitochondrial oxidative phosphorylation and aerobic glycolysis [13, 15]. Given the ability of MitoQ to accumulate at large concentrations in the mitochondria [3], it is not altogether surprising that MitoQ has a profound effect on the viability of cells with increased mitochondrial respiratory capacities. In summary, more research is needed to investigate molecular vulnerabilities among these subgroups.

Acknowledgements

This work was supported by research grants from the American Cancer Society Research Scholar Grant 120634-RSG-11-269-01-CDD and the Georgia Research Alliance. We appreciate Brian S. Cummings for providing helpful discussions and thank Pooya Hoseinzadeh for assistance in the laboratory.

http://dx.doi.org/10.5772/64231

Author details

Ali A. Alshamrani, James L. Franklin, Aaron M. Beedle and Mandi M. Murph*

*Address all correspondence to: mmurph@uga.edu

Department of Pharmaceutical and Biomedical Sciences, College of Pharmacy, The University of Georgia, Athens, GA, United States of America

References

[1] Murphy MP: Selective targeting of bioactive compounds to mitochondria. Trend Biotechnol 1997, 15(8):326–330.

[2] Cocheme HM, Kelso GF, James AM, Ross MF, Trnka J, Mahendiran T, Asin-Cayuela J, Blaikie FH, Manas AR, Porteous CM et al: Mitochondrial targeting of quinones: therapeutic implications. Mitochondrion 2007, 7(Suppl):S94–S102.

[3] Murphy MP, Smith RA: Targeting antioxidants to mitochondria by conjugation to lipophilic cations. Annu Rev Pharmacol Toxicol 2007, 47:629–656.

[4] Kelso GF, Porteous CM, Coulter CV, Hughes G, Porteous WK, Ledgerwood EC, Smith RA, Murphy MP: Selective targeting of a redox-active ubiquinone to mitochondria within cells: antioxidant and antiapoptotic properties. J Biol Chem 2001, 276(7):4588–4596.

[5] Trnka J, Elkalaf M, Andel M: Lipophilic triphenylphosphonium cations inhibit mitochondrial electron transport chain and induce mitochondrial proton leak. PLoS One 2015, 10(4):e0121837.

[6] Gonzalez Y, Aryal B, Chehab L, Rao VA: Atg7- and Keap1-dependent autophagy protects breast cancer cell lines against mitoquinone-induced oxidative stress. Oncotarget 2014, 5(6):1526–1537.

[7] Dilip A, Cheng G, Joseph J, Kunnimalaiyaan S, Kalyanaraman B, Kunnimalaiyaan M, Gamblin TC: Mitochondria-targeted antioxidant and glycolysis inhibition: synergistic therapy in hepatocellular carcinoma. Anticancer Drugs 2013, 24(9):881–888.

[8] Cheng G, Zielonka J, Dranka BP, McAllister D, Mackinnon AC Jr., Joseph J, Kalyanaraman B: Mitochondria-targeted drugs synergize with 2-deoxyglucose to trigger breast cancer cell death. Cancer Res 2012, 72(10):2634–2644.

[9] Smith RA, Murphy MP: Animal and human studies with the mitochondria-targeted antioxidant MitoQ. Ann N Y Acad Sci 2010, 1201:96–103.

[10] Oyewole AO, Birch-Machin MA: Mitochondria-targeted antioxidants. FASEB J 2015, 29(12):4766–4771.

[11] Warburg O: On respiratory impairment in cancer cells. Science 1956, 124(3215):269–270.

[12] Hanahan D, Weinberg RA: Hallmarks of cancer: the next generation. Cell 2011, 144(5): 646–674.

[13] Haq R, Fisher DE, Widlund HR: Molecular pathways: BRAF induces bioenergetic adaptation by attenuating oxidative phosphorylation. Clin Cancer Res 2014, 20(9):2257–2263.

[14] Theodosakis N, Micevic G, Kelly DP, Bosenberg M: Mitochondrial function in melanoma. Arch Biochem Biophys 2014, 563:56–59.

[15] Abildgaard C, Guldberg P: Molecular drivers of cellular metabolic reprogramming in melanoma. Trends Mol Med 2015, 21(3):164–171.

[16] Marroquin LD, Hynes J, Dykens JA, Jamieson JD, Will Y: Circumventing the Crabtree effect: replacing media glucose with galactose increases susceptibility of HepG2 cells to mitochondrial toxicants. Toxicol Sci 2007, 97(2):539–547.

[17] Hasegawa Y, Murph M, Yu S, Tigyi G, Mills GB: Lysophosphatidic acid (LPA)-induced vasodilator-stimulated phosphoprotein mediates lamellipodia formation to initiate motility in PC-3 prostate cancer cells. Mol Oncol 2008, 2(1):54–69.

[18] Altman MK, Gopal V, Jia W, Yu S, Hall H, Mills GB, McGinnis AC, Bartlett MG, Jiang G, Madan D et al: Targeting melanoma growth and viability reveals dualistic functionality of the phosphonothionate analogue of carba cyclic phosphatidic acid. Mol Cancer 2010, 9:140.

[19] Hooks SB, Callihan P, Altman MK, Hurst JH, Ali MW, Murph MM: Regulators of G-Protein signaling RGS10 and RGS17 regulate chemoresistance in ovarian cancer cells. Mol Cancer 2010, 9:289.

[20] Murph MM, Jiang GW, Altman MK, Jia W, Nguyen DT, Fambrough JM, Hardman WJ, Nguyen HT, Tran SK, Alshamrani AA et al: Vinyl sulfone analogs of lysophosphatidylcholine irreversibly inhibit autotaxin and prevent angiogenesis in melanoma. Bioorg Med Chem. 2015 Sep 1;23(17):5999–6013.

[21] Rossignol R, Gilkerson R, Aggeler R, Yamagata K, Remington SJ, Capaldi RA: Energy substrate modulates mitochondrial structure and oxidative capacity in cancer cells. Cancer Res 2004, 64(3):985–993.

[22] Dykens JA, Jamieson J, Marroquin L, Nadanaciva S, Billis PA, Will Y: Biguanide-induced mitochondrial dysfunction yields increased lactate production and cytotoxicity of aerobically-poised HepG2 cells and human hepatocytes in vitro. Toxicol Appl Pharmacol 2008, 233(2):203–210.

[23] Rana P, Nadanaciva S, Will Y: Mitochondrial membrane potential measurement of H9c2 cells grown in high-glucose and galactose-containing media does not provide addi-

tional predictivity towards mitochondrial assessment. Toxicol In Vitro 2011, 25(2):580–587.

[24] Zhao Y, Butler EB, Tan M: Targeting cellular metabolism to improve cancer therapeutics. Cell Death Dis 2013, 4:e532.

[25] Zhuang L, Scolyer RA, Murali R, McCarthy SW, Zhang XD, Thompson JF, Hersey P: Lactate dehydrogenase 5 expression in melanoma increases with disease progression and is associated with expression of Bcl-XL and Mcl-1, but not Bcl-2 proteins. Mod Pathol 2010, 23(1):45–53.

[26] Doherty JR, Cleveland JL: Targeting lactate metabolism for cancer therapeutics. J Clin Invest 2013, 123(9):3685–3692.

[27] O'Day SJ, Eggermont AM, Chiarion-Sileni V, Kefford R, Grob JJ, Mortier L, Robert C, Schachter J, Testori A, Mackiewicz J et al: Final results of phase III SYMMETRY study: randomized, double-blind trial of elesclomol plus paclitaxel versus paclitaxel alone as treatment for chemotherapy-naive patients with advanced melanoma. J Clin Oncol 2013, 31(9):1211–1218.

[28] Cheng G, Zielonka J, McAllister DM, Mackinnon AC, Jr., Joseph J, Dwinell MB, Kalyanaraman B: Mitochondria-targeted vitamin E analogs inhibit breast cancer cell energy metabolism and promote cell death. BMC Cancer 2013, 13:285.

[29] Baker DL, Fujiwara Y, Pigg KR, Tsukahara R, Kobayashi S, Murofushi H, Uchiyama A, Murakami-Murofushi K, Koh E, Bandle RW et al: Carba analogs of cyclic phosphatidic acid are selective inhibitors of autotaxin and cancer cell invasion and metastasis. J Biol Chem 2006, 281(32):22786–22793.

[30] Samadi N, Gaetano C, Goping IS, Brindley DN: Autotaxin protects MCF-7 breast cancer and MDA-MB-435 melanoma cells against Taxol-induced apoptosis. Oncogene 2009, 28(7):1028–1039.

[31] Vazquez F, Lim JH, Chim H, Bhalla K, Girnun G, Pierce K, Clish CB, Granter SR, Widlund HR, Spiegelman BM et al: PGC1alpha expression defines a subset of human melanoma tumors with increased mitochondrial capacity and resistance to oxidative stress. Cancer Cell 2013, 23(3):287–301.

[32] Cancer Genome Atlas N: Genomic classification of cutaneous melanoma. Cell 2015, 161(7):1681–1696.